SEASONS OF GRIEF

by the same author

The Creative Toolkit for Working with Grief and Bereavement
A Practitioner's Guide with Activities and Worksheets
Claudia Coenen
Illustrated by Masha Pimas
ISBN 978 1 78775 146 0
eISBN 978 1 78775 147 7

Shattered by Grief
Picking up the pieces to become WHOLE again
Claudia Coenen
ISBN 978 1 78592 777 5
eISBN 978 1 78450 695 7

Karuna Cards
Creative Ideas to Transform Grief and Difficult Life Transitions
Claudia Coenen
ISBN 978 1 78592 780 5

of related interest

Creative Counselling
Creative Tools and Interventions to Nurture Therapeutic Relationships
Tanja Sharpe
Foreword by Suzanne Alderson
ISBN 978 1 83997 018 4
eISBN 978 1 83997 017 7

Supporting Your Grieving Client
A Guide for Wellness Practitioners
Vanessa May
ISBN 978 1 83997 347 5
eISBN 978 1 83997 348 2

Seasons of Grief

Creative Interventions to Support Bereaved People

Edited by Claudia Coenen

Foreword by Kenneth J. Doka, PhD

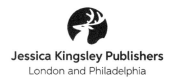

Jessica Kingsley Publishers
London and Philadelphia

First published in Great Britain in 2024 by Jessica Kingsley Publishers
An imprint of John Murray Press

2

A CIP catalogue record for this title is available from the British Library and the Library of Congress

ISBN 978 1 83997 486 1
eISBN 978 1 83997 487 8

Printed and bound by CPI Group (UK) Ltd, Croydon, CR0 4YY

Jessica Kingsley Publishers' policy is to use papers that are natural, renewable and recyclable products and made from wood grown in sustainable forests. The logging and manufacturing processes are expected to conform to the environmental regulations of the country of origin.

Jessica Kingsley Publishers
Carmelite House
50 Victoria Embankment
London EC4Y 0DZ

www.jkp.com

John Murray Press
Part of Hodder & Stoughton Ltd
An Hachette Company

Contents

Preface

Claudia Coenen

A seed sprouts, deep in the forest. Over time, it becomes a large tree. It provides shade, shelter, food, homes for animals. Every autumn, the leaves burst into color, then shrivel up and fall. The tree is bare in the cold winter, its branches splayed gracefully against the sky like multi-fingered hands dancing in the breeze. In spring, the earth and air warm, stimulating the lifeblood of tree sap, generating new leaves and more growth. This cycle repeats itself until the tree dies, falling and collapsing on the forest floor. As it rots, it becomes nutrients, supplying energy for mushrooms to grow, hollows for animals to burrow. The tree disintegrates into earth, allowing its cells to enrich the soil from which new little trees will sprout.

Life follows a similar path, unfolding from birth in what seems like a linear progression of time. We are born, hopefully are sheltered, nurtured and encouraged to grow. We have relationships and achievements. We learn, fail, make friends, expand our families. If we are lucky, we live a full life before we die. For those of us left behind, we mourn, grieve and slowly learn how to live with our grief and our loss. This book contains stories of how others have managed that, with musings, personal examples, case studies and clinical interventions from professional practitioners who work with grieving people. There are specific techniques that you can use for your own grief and for those bereaved people you might encounter. There are poems, art, reflections and photographs of the interventions themselves.

My own life has always flowed on waves of creativity, since I was a child. The movement of trees in the wind would inspire me to twirl and leap. A longing to understand love and connection inspired me to read incessantly and to listen deeply to old ballads, classical music and jazz. Music contained emotions that lingered between the lines of a song or appeared in an image evoked by the distillation of a poetic phrase. My body pulsed with the need to express these feelings, and I made many dances which did just that. My early fascination with mythology led me to try to sense the energy beneath the surface of ordinary life; for me, this is where we discover meaning. Looking back over time, I see disruptions and stoppages that tossed me off the trajectory I thought I was following. Upheaval, loss, death and, of course, grief—the sea of life is not smooth or predictable. The tumultuous and difficult parts of life offer choice points: we can collapse and disintegrate on the forest floor, or we can dissolve into something more nutritious, something that helps us discover new meaning in the midst of the devastation. While grief requires us to wallow inside it for a while, there is much to learn in the process of discovery. How is it possible to be alive when so much has been lost? How can we gather up the remnants of love and connection we shared and carry them with us as we plant new seeds?

Ancient peoples measured their lives around seasons, weather, the phases of the moon and other celestial observances, developing mythologies and beliefs that explained the natural phenomena according to their culture and the place in which they lived, hunted, gathered and made homes.

In ancient Celtic tradition and in others, communities celebrated solstices and equinoxes as well as cross-quarter points. People imagined these times to be both powerful and fragile, cracking open the space between the physical world and the liminal. The Celts celebrated Samhain, or All Hallows, when the barrier between life and death cracks open. This is also El Día de los Muertos in Hispanic cultures, when families picnic with their ancestors on top of their graves and place offerings on a shrine called an ofrenda, with photographs of ancestors and treats for them to eat. Halloween, often celebrated with costumes and candy, was originally a response to this thinning of the veil. In early February, in the deepest winter in the North, there is the cross point of Candlemas. Here, in the darkest, most internal time, deep beneath the ground, seeds are stirring. New life opens in the darkness. Beltane or May Day celebrates the burgeoning of spring, and people traditionally dance around a maypole, weaving brightly colored ribbons down its tall shaft, laughing as they tried to remember whether to go over or under to create the braid. Lammas is an August celebration, when the fruits of the harvest are gathered to nurture us all. These cardinal points in the year correspond to the cycle of the seasons and the activities of people during each one, whether it is a growing season, a harvest season or the time of rest and rejuvenation.

When we survive the death of a beloved person, pet or activity that fulfilled us and gave meaning to our lives, we grieve and mourn, but we also come to understand that we might find a way to rise from the devastation. While transformation is a tricky proposition, especially for those who suffer the death of a child or are struggling in the aftermath of a homicide or suicide, if we view our grief through the lens of the seasons, we can be guided towards slowly beginning to live again. We discover new ways to remain connected to those who are no longer physically here, and we create purpose in our lives after loss. To me, that is a definition of transformation.

As spiritually skeptical as I am in many ways, it was the death of my husband that gave me permission to let go of some of the questions about what is "true" and what cannot be empirically verified. I have always sought the "why" of things, and while this has set me on a path of inquiry and learning, death taught me there are some questions that have no answers. We do not know *why* someone dies when they do. We might blame cancer, or a doctor who didn't diagnose it in time. We might blame bad weather for a car accident, or alcohol or drugs. We might say that a person's lifestyle set up conditions that caused illness, a stroke or a heart attack, but we do not really know the answer. Some even blame negative thinking for disease and tell people with terminal illness that they can cure themselves if they just think a different way. No amount of explaining or blaming can answer "Why?" The last thing a grieving person needs to hear is that they should have known the answer to this unanswerable question.

Why does one person live to be 100 and another die at 23 or 7? Why does a person who has no regard for others live and seemingly thrive when another who was kind dies young? What is the answer to why someone takes a military-grade rifle into a school to mow down children? We can blame bad parenting, poverty, mental illness, political inaction, but really we do not know. We can only find our way through the devastation and figure out how to cope and live with the loss. This is not easy; the emotions of grief are dysregulating and huge. They seem to interrupt the flow of our lives and bring us to our knees. Sitting in the rubble of our assumptions, it is hard to imagine the years ahead. How will we get up? How will we reshape our shattered world?

We have inner resources available to us even when we feel lost and broken. We can seek help from a friend, a counselor or advisor who has loved and lost. Perhaps this person has used their own life experience of wreckage and repair and studied how others have managed. Through experience, experimentation, insight and serendipity, wise guides are available to share what they have learned, to help you rise from the shards of loss. Their ideas and suggestions will help you discover your own path through loss and will guide you towards finding ways to assist and companion others in their grief.

I view life through a creative lens. Creativity flowered when I was a musician, a dancer and choreographer. Creativity is present in the way that I cook, combining herbs and spices, vegetables and proteins to create delicious and beautiful nourishment. I have done this for my family and friends, and for hundreds of guests at dinner parties, celebrations and weddings that I catered. Keeping the connection alive and love flowing in my close relationships often requires a creative approach. The work I engage in now, counseling deeply bereaved people who are struggling to get through the day, is assisted by creativity, whether it arises in a metaphor, a collage, a drawing, movement or retelling their story in a different way.

This book brings together a group of wise heart-centered therapists with different viewpoints. It includes a doula, a music thanatologist, a playwright whose work stimulates conversation about death and dying, a former graphic designer who now helps people with different abilities find work. The group also contains researchers, professors, psychologists, educators. Viewpoints come from art therapy, constructivist, transpersonal, somatic, nature-based and yoga therapy as well as personal experiences of the writers.

We gathered in Zoom Wisdom Circles to share our progress, joining together upon the ground of grief and creativity. We have learned through experience that trauma, loss and death shape us in many ways. We each have our own styles, personal and professional perspectives, and our own voices, but we all agree that creativity provides an open field on which to express, understand and grow through grief. Jean Houston says:

> Everyone of us is a roiling cauldron of creative process. It's just that we haven't developed the hooks and eyes to catch the creative idea as it emerges. But that doesn't mean it can't happen. Do you hear what I am saying? Wherever there is an impetus, the passion, the yearning that reaches a certain point of passionate possibility, you will tend to do it. (Houston, 2008)

This book offers techniques to stimulate that creative process. Grief is so huge, so all-encompassing that it longs for release. Expressive modalities provide just that. As Ken Doka says, it is natural and cathartic, "releasing pent-up energy as you engage in the activity" (Doka, 2016).

Everyone writing in this book lives in the Northern Hemisphere, and you may live in another part of the world. We acknowledge that when we are in the deep of winter, you might be enjoying summers at the beach. We invite you to apply these techniques to your own environment. We are also aware that there may be cultural differences, and if some of these have not been adequately acknowledged, we wish you to know that we have tried to be sensitive to them. You may find spelling differences within these pages since there is a difference between American and British spellings. We have left them alone in honor (honour!) of each writer's own place. It is our intention to be inclusive of unique perspectives, culture, origins and how each writer authentically express themselves. We will all experience grief; those of us writing for this book are actively and compassionately here to listen, to *be* with our clients, our friends and colleagues and anyone struggling through personal grief as well as the collective grief of the world in this strange time.

One contributor, Louise Allen, is an integrative counselor in Kent, England. She shared her evocative description of the burgeoning growth of forest and field, followed by the subsequent dying and disintegration, which reflects the cycle of life and love. Louise inspired me to shape this book through a seasonal lens. Dr. Robert A. Neimeyer offered the phrases framing each season and three of his beautiful poems open Parts One, Two and Three for Autumn, Winter and Spring. Deborah Mesibov, a dear friend, has been writing poetry for years and her poem about her father, Hugh Mesibov, who was a respected American artist, prolific until his death at almost 100 years old, opens Part Four: Summer. Another old friend, Steven "Mud" Roues, is an accomplished musician and poet who has, like all of us, experienced many losses in his life. His poems are sprinkled here and there.

Contributors placed their chapters in the season that felt most aligned with the intervention they were offering. Of course, we know that you can use these ideas and techniques in any season since one does not only journal in winter or enjoy nature in summer. The seasonal lens is a construct to allow us to explore grief and the cycle of life metaphorically. I hope you will be inspired by the creativity expressed in the images, poetry and techniques. May they help you with your own grief and the bereaved people you encounter and perhaps work with.

Deborah Koff-Chapin's evocative Touch Drawings frame each season and appear throughout the book. She writes about her art in Chapter 9. The images in this book were chosen from thousands of drawings she has made over the years; they are a reminder that viewing imagery opens intuitive paths in the heart, mind and body. I invite you to sit with any of the images in this book and allow yourself to respond to them.

Looking through a seasonal lens, the natural world becomes a symbol for our own inner world and a metaphor for healing. Louise Allen explains this in her own words:

> I see the other-than-human world around me as equal in the therapeutic process as a counsellor and for the people I counsel. We are in a continually evolving relationship; the person having counselling, myself as counsellor and nature. I look to psychotherapy theory and the human experience for inspiration, and I look to nature to learn how we might live, grieve, grow and die in the fullest and most authentic way possible. In nature, we have commonalities and differences and our own ways of living and protecting ourselves. We have our own yearnings and directions we want to grow, and our own ways of experiencing pain, joy, love and loss.
>
> Just as the emotional, physical and social conditions we grow up in inform and shape our inner selves, the way we develop as people can often be reflected in wider nature. From the way we build society, our homes, the way we interact with others, to the way we feel inside—these processes inform the ways we protect, nurture or create the conditions in which to grow and thrive. Our inner worlds are as complex as the outer world we exist within.
>
> Cycles can be observed in the natural processes around and within us. The seasons, the lunar cycle, the tides, menstruation, reproduction, spiral us out (blossoming) into adults and spiral us in towards death, composting, leaving legacies in some form or another.
>
> We exist within these cycles, and we choose or are thrown into lifestyles that sometimes align, sometimes clash with these. At the same time, our own inner seasons are happening, our energy levels ebbing and flowing; taking in information, processing, considering what to do with it, putting it out/creating/producing with what we have absorbed. We see these cycles in our patterns of behaviour, in our relationships, in our education and career paths, in our aspirations.
>
> We may not always feel aligned internally with the external weather or seasons—perhaps we are going through a divorce or feeling the desolation

of grief during summer when birds are singing and flowers are in full bloom. We may draw inspiration, learning and perhaps comfort from acknowledging that, like the rest of nature, we too go through cycles and no feeling lasts forever.

I invite you to enter the seasons of grief with us. Feel free to move around and read in any order you wish. Life is a cycle, grief itself is cyclical as it curves and spirals around itself. Creativity can carry us on the cusp of a wave, and if we tumble down to the bottom of a dark abyss of sadness, creative process will guide us out.

References

Doka, K.J. (2016). *Grief Is a Journey: Finding Your Path through Loss*. New York, NY: Atria Paperback.

Houston, J. (2008). *Wise Women in a Wild Wild World*. Seattle, WA: Wise Women Publishing.

In the days following the death, it can feel as if the beach you know so well is disappearing before your eyes. As the sea recedes, just as it does at the start of a tsunami, your beach may become unrecognizable to you and you are not sure what is happening to you...

Gradually you find yourself able to muster the energy to clear a path through the flotsam and jetsam of your desolated beach. You are becoming more familiar with the contours of the shifting sands. A way forward gradually begins to appear. You may find yourself moving forward on this path but at times turning back to the beach again.

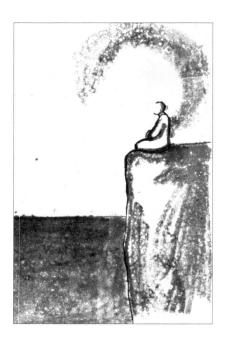

Surviving the Tsunami of Grief by Katrina Taee and Wendelien McNicoll

Foreword

Kenneth J. Doka, PhD, Senior Vice-President, The Hospice Foundation of America Professor Emeritus, The College of New Rochelle

For most of my educational career, I was privileged to teach at the Graduate School of the College of New Rochelle. My students came from a variety of programs—graduate nursing, guidance and counseling, school psychology, mental health counseling, gerontology, and art therapy. Some of my students were seasoned professionals—already possessing an advanced degree but wishing to obtain a Certificate in Grief Counseling (Thanatology). This led to an incredibly rich exchange, and I hoped (and thought) a great deal of mutual learning.

As I think about this book, I am reminded of two lessons.

The first one was a negative lesson. One of my Certificate students was a seasoned yet very dogmatic expressively oriented therapist who thought molding with clay was the ultimate and only tool one needed. Her answer to "What approach might you use in this case?" was resoundingly and uniformly "Clay." No matter how much we agreed that clay could be a useful instrument in the therapist's toolkit, to her it was the only modality necessary. Even when students pointed out that, for some of them, the feel of clay was clammy and unpleasant, she dismissed them. Yet the first principle of expressive therapy is that no modality works for everyone all the time.

The second experience was much more positive. When I was five years old, I sustained a bad break in my dominant right arm. Even after four operations and physical therapy, I never regained full use. So I became left-handed. But as a convert to left-handedness, I lacked fine motor coordination. Hence, I never liked art classes or even arts and crafts at camp. At camp, I would even not show up at arts and crafts but instead look for sanctuary at the Nature Hut. The camp director did not want to make an issue of it—camp was, after all, to be a fun experience. Instead, he directed the Nature Counselor to try to gently discourage my presence by having me clean the cages of the varied creatures and reptiles represented there. That, he reasoned, would quickly encourage my return to arts and crafts.

It didn't work. I loved cleaning the cages. I was able to pick up and hold all of the fascinating creatures and even lost any residual fear of snakes I might have had. I joked with my students that if I ever entered a nursing home—aged and with dementia—that they should not wheel me into arts and crafts. The last thing I would ever forget was that I hated it. I reminded them that even at seven years of age, given the choice of arts and crafts or cleaning snake crap, I happily selected the latter! I concluded that other expressive therapies such as storytelling were far better approaches for me than art therapy.

One of my art therapy students challenged me—insisting that she could employ art approaches that would engage me. I accepted her challenge sure that I would win.

I lost. She had me do all sorts of interesting art projects such as spin art, finger painting—even sand art. All were tied to grief, and none required that fine motor coordination.

So I learned another lesson about expressive therapies. Applied in a very individual manner, almost any approach can succeed.

Expressive approaches work because they are natural. They are a common and creative activity to express what is being experienced. Whether it is writing poetry, journaling or writing short stories, music, dancing or other body movements, storytelling, art, or any other expressive approach, we all have a creative side.

These approaches are reflective—allowing us to explore our creations. And sometimes we gain new insights about ourselves as our unconscious self can find expression.

These approaches are cathartic—releasing pent-up energy as you engage in the activity. Our anger can be released in the furious movements of our dance or our drawings. Our sadness is released in what we write and sing. In grief, the products of our activity can even be a legacy to the love now lost—witness Eric Clapton's memorial song for his son: "Tears in Heaven."

They draw from your inner self—connecting you to your culture, background, and beliefs. The modalities we use and the symbols represented there draw from our background and past experiences. They emphasize rather than ignore our individuality.

Finally, and most importantly, they work.

The great strength of this book is that it reaffirms both the value and the importance of individuality of expressive therapies. The book offers a treasure of expressive approaches—a venerable toolbox of techniques. It will be a classic—a book that every therapist will want on his or her shelf—to be often consulted.

PART ONE

AUTUMN

Letting Go

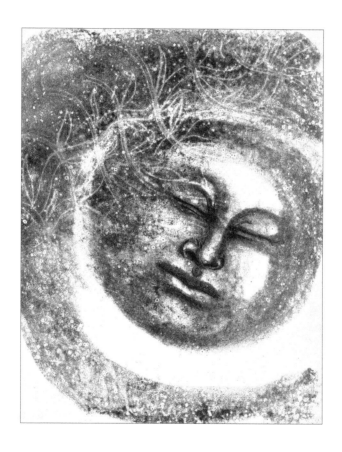

Falls

At water's edge
the liquid silence pools, deepens,
readies for the plunge.

Slipping over, it atomizes,
pearls in droplets
promiscuous in their
joining and letting go.

In that long fall,
free as doves bursting into
flight, they ride the roar,
crash to earth,
rejoin the
whole.

Above,
moored at the abyss,
I ride the mist
like a wave,
sense the stillness,
and ready myself

for the plunge.

~ Robert A. Neimeyer

Autumn Reflection

Claudia Coenen

In autumn, we let go of the activities that kept us going all summer. Flowers die back, leaves change color, turn brown and shrivel up, falling to the earth in piles and heaps. My grief is like this too. It changes and dries up, it fills the corners of my mind with piles of memories, items left over from the life that is no longer. In the season of the fall, I realize that I too have fallen to the earth. I can do nothing but lie on my back, staring up at the sky through the trees that are slowly baring their branches.

This is a time of reflection on what has passed, on what is slipping away. As air crisps and we reach for a sweater or shawl and a hat to keep us warm, we realize that we must loosen our grip. We cannot hold back the change of seasons; we cannot touch the ones who have died. Slowly, we begin to slide into our internal world. The shriveling of everything around us is sensed inside our bodies. What is dying off now? What do I need to release? How shall I relinquish what is no longer present, that I still long for but can no longer keep? Shall I carry my grief, in its bucket of raw pain, into the interior of my body? Or is there another place I can keep it, tending to its needs, listening to its wail, enveloping it in warmth so it can be soothed?

I have poured grief into a chalice of my pain and my ended relationship. It is enclosed within the thin walls of this container—which looks like a golden ewer, wider at the bottom, tapering into a graceful waist and opening at the top with a small spout. The handle has a slight curl at its base where it joins the chalice. Contained, narrowing, tapering and opening, its curve fits in my palm as I raise the chalice.

I lift the chalice and look for a place to pour my grief. Then I put it back down again.

Grief will wait. Perhaps I should explore what moving away from grief feels like. There is plenty of time. It is not going anywhere.

Letting go of holding my grief all the time, of pouring it over me again and again, I begin to ask a different question than "Where do I put my grief?" I begin to ask myself, "What is next?" What is arising, on the horizon, in the world, in my own psyche? What is arising in my heart?

I sit next to the chalice, gazing out. I do not know what is next, but I am open to it. I am ready.

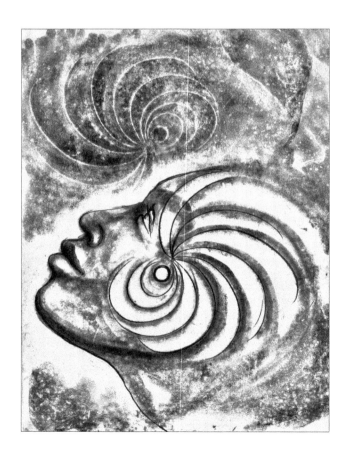

CHAPTER 1

Letting Go and Room to Grow

Louise Allen

Introduction

M y therapeutic work is heavily inspired by nature and woven together with what we understand of our conscious awareness of our existence and mortality. In a culture where we are so often disconnected from much of our nature, where we live within structures that control and manage and defend against the rest of nature, I find wisdom and freedom in the therapeutic accept-

Perhaps a closed oyster shell represents how someone feels about beginning a new relationship after the death of a partner. They may see the layers of protection in the shell. Perhaps a vulnerable, broken heart is the pearl within.

ance of natural life cycles and processes, the relatedness of plants and animals, how the weather and seasons can be so reminiscent of our internal processes.

Working in a nature-inspired way can be indoors, outdoors and remote. The nature-inspired interventions I have included in this book focus on working outdoors but can mostly be adapted in a variety of settings. One of the benefits of working outdoors is that, although we may not always explicitly bring in observations of what we see or are taking from the woodland or the sea, for example, it continues around us regardless and we sense it and are part of it. Just as our experience in grief is continually evolving, complex and in relation to other people, environments, smells, hopes, memories, so it is to be human with our full range of human emotions, and so the more of this we can hold space for in therapy, the richer, broader and deeper the experience may be.

Many people find being with other-than-human nature a way of feeling free to feel and be without fear of judgement—whether that be through throwing stones into a river, stroking a dog or walking among the trees. The natural world becomes a space of non-judgement and acceptance. Taking the empathic and compassionate therapist/client relationship into nature gently nurtures the client/nature relationship as a one of healing where nature can become a constant source of continuation, unpredictable but always there in some way. However, it is important to be mindful that for those who have had traumatic or negative experiences outdoors, or who have been cut off and disconnected in their relationship with their outer world, their relationship with nature may be less positive or potentially re-traumatising. With this in mind, to collaboratively assess suitability for outdoor therapy, I'd recommend getting to know someone and discussing their relationship with nature and the other-than-human and human beings you may come into contact with when working outdoors. This might be dogs, passers-by, different weather conditions and particular areas you might meet. This helps begin to set a relational and psychological grounding for holding what comes into an unpredictable physical space.

As with all therapeutic approaches, when working outdoors, it is important to work within one's competencies and ensure that any new or different risks and opportunities for psychological processes are understood. There are a growing number of outdoor therapy, walking therapy and ecotherapy courses and workshops to ensure you have a good grounding in working ethically outdoors. I'd recommend an experiential workshop as working outdoors can feel very different. As well as emotional and physical safety, there are issues around boundaries, power, accessibility, disclosure and privacy to consider. Practical considerations around preparing for sessions, allergies, routes and what to do in an emergency are also essential. You will also want to check how and if your insurance provider covers outdoor working.

To introduce each of the techniques or interventions, I offer some of my own nature-inspired journey that has informed my use of them. Each journey may include some knowledge about the other-than-human world along with my own way of communicating what I observe. It is important to me to acknowledge that I am continually growing and becoming, and I strive to maintain an open position of not knowing and learning from the people I counsel, myself and wider nature. I share these interventions with the awareness that you and your clients may have a different relationship to the natural world, and will most likely have further observations and knowledge to weave in. I hope that you find some inspiration from the interventions.

Change and transition can be seen around us all year round if we are paying attention, but autumn's vibrancy really calls for us to take notice of the transition process and loss. What we know and understand about other-than-human and more-than-human nature is, of course, wildly varied from person to person and culture to culture. Perhaps you are a botanist or zoologist able to identify hundreds of species, perhaps you spend hours each week walking one particular stretch of beach and know it intimately, perhaps you like looking at the shapes and movement of the trees out of the window but haven't given their species' names much thought. We observe, think, sense and emote in relation to nature, and these aspects all contribute to our experience. In autumn, I notice that there is a busyness of preparation for the longer nights and the colder temperatures. An abundance of berries, nuts and fruit, which I know to be full of fats and sugars and so can sustain animal life through the scarcity of winter. I feel excited by the changing colours and the pull towards cosying up. What does autumn mean to you? What do you observe of autumn? How do you feel within autumn?

In autumn, the leaves of deciduous trees change colour as the daylight hours and temperature change. Just as we change emotionally, psychologically and behaviourally in reaction to the conditions around us, enabling us to survive. I have learnt that the leaves are green with chlorophyll pigment during the warmer, brighter months, using the sun's energy to make food for the tree. In autumn, as there is less sunlight, the chlorophyll breaks down, revealing the yellow and orange hues of carotenoids—pigments that were there all along, but covered up by the prominent green in summer. A vibrant metaphor for how the changes in our social, physical and economic environment reveal different layers, different aspects of us and other beings. In some trees, like maples, we also see the reds and purples of anthocyanins—pigment formed by sunlight converting the sugar trapped in the leaves. Different from a revealing of what was already there, we see alchemy, a conversion into something new. Both processes are inherently based in the interconnectedness of beings and the conditions in which they exist.

When we are aware of a change occurring, or having occurred, it confronts us with an awareness of change in itself—of things not always being as they currently are. This awareness of what was and what will, might or will not be means we can be taken away from the present moment. This is a sometimes helpful, sometimes hindering paradigm that disengages us from our current feelings and experience. When our present feelings are uncomfortable, painful or harmful, we can imagine our way out of the present, longing to be at a stage we are not currently at. This can feel frustrating, tedious, overwhelming, desperate, hopeless, demoralising, exhausting, depressing, scary. It can feel as if we will be stuck in the situation or feeling or psychological dynamic forever. One autumn, when I was going through a period of painful personal loss, the changes felt painstakingly slow, an almost oxymoron of relentless stasis. Walking through fallen maple leaves, I realised I was thinking, "It's still autumn! I have been walking through fallen leaves for ages," and I had an acute sense that I couldn't do anything about it. I needed to acknowledge my frustration and desperation—autumn leaves are quite wonderful for trudging, stomping and kicking through! Gradually, I was able to see the little changes. There were more leaves on the ground. There were leaves still changing colour. I thought then, "I'm still in autumn. There are leaves I'm walking through. Some are new; this is how they look. Some have been here a while; this is how they look now. Perhaps more will fall. Perhaps the weather will change. I wonder what I will notice then." Noticing the movement, the tiny changes, was both painful and reassuring. It reminded me that it will not be this way forever, and stretching out my awareness opened up space for me to hold my frustration, exhaustion, sadness alongside the beauty and stillness, the acknowledgement of where I wanted to be, what had been before and where I was.

I share some journal prompts below. Inspired by the changing colours of the leaves, these prompts may be useful for processing the awareness of change. Used in between therapy sessions or following a session where a shift or change has been identified, these prompts may help to broaden the person's awareness of the impact of the changes.

As a therapist, you may find these prompts valuable in nurturing your own relationship with other-than-human nature as you explore similarities in your own process of change with those of the trees around you. This might also be an insightful self-supervision exercise for you as a therapist to explore the ending of work with a client.

Journal Prompts

Think of a loss in your life. It could be the death of someone close to you, the end of a relationship, moving home or changing job, for example. You might like to imagine you are a deciduous tree, with the changing conditions around you representing your loss or the change in your life.

- What did this change reveal of you? What parts of you—your long-ings, hopes, emotions, identity, strengths, vulnerabilities, beliefs, etc.—emerged through the process?
- Did anything change within you as life around you changed?
- Draw what you looked like (as a tree) before the loss, and then after.

I sometimes imagine our inner world as lush, wild vegetation and animal life, available for exploration if we dare. I am drawn to the imagery of a fid-dlehead fern, emerging tender and coiled, gradually unfurling and opening into fullness. And, as with the fern, sometimes parts of us, or ways of being, die back. This makes space for new growth. We are all going through per-sonal transitions all the time. We are also all part of a wider ecosystem and are interconnected with many other transitions in nature, both human and more-than- or other-than-human.

Therapy or counselling is a space both to unfurl and understand how the conditions of our inner and outer worlds affect our growth, and to un-derstand what has or needs to die back to allow for this. It can be a space to be with what it is like when something in us or someone connected to us dies. To bear witness to and allow the cycle of growth and death within and around us. To understand what impact that has on our inner ecosystem and the fullness of the emotions that come up. The following intervention is an exploration of the transition process, inviting the person to take inspiration from the richness of their external natural world, to explore and understand their experience of the changes they are going through.

It offers an opportunity to explore where they are, and how the different parts of themselves and the process relate. It can be broad or acute in focus depending on the person's need and preference. It gives an opportunity to both be inspired by and learn from nature, and/or work with nature as a metaphor to convey a personal experience.

The intervention is inspired by the often-cyclical transitions in other-than-human nature and our relationship with them, and it is adapted from the ChrisLin Method and framework of questioning. The technique is a process of creative enquiry which invites us to represent and communicate the story of our transition, exploring the relationship between the different components. It is based on the idea that there are four components to a transition in which we may feel "stuck." These are:

- There is not a big enough reason for *why* the change should happen.
- Building up all the things I don't want to let go of.
- Fear of making a mistake/getting it wrong.
- Doesn't feel like a choice.

Preparation

This can be done online, on the phone, indoors or outdoors. What you need to prepare for the session will depend on where you are meeting.

This intervention tends to take a whole 50–60-minute session (or even longer). In my experience, planning the session in advance together with the person is helpful, rather than bringing it in reflexively midway through a session.

If you are meeting online, you will need images of different places or beings in nature—woods, the beach, birds, trees, nests, mountains, etc. Decide in advance who will source and share the images on the screen. You might want to find a selection and share them for the person to look through and choose from. Or they might want to find an image (or images) that represents their transition before the session.

If you are working on the telephone, the person will need images or a view of nature that represent their transition. This might be the view of fields from their window, a house plant, photos on a computer or from a magazine, or a painting.

If you are working indoors, you might like to source a selection of nature imagery cards (such as *The Wild Cards*[1]) or cut some photos from magazines. You could have a wide selection of animals, plants, landscapes and seasons so that the person can create their own collage with different components to represent their transition. Or they may have their own photo or image to bring.

If you work outdoors in a way that means you have a choice of where you meet for your sessions, you might want to invite the person to choose the

---

[1] *The Wild Cards* by Robert McFarlane and Jackie Morris (Hamish Hamilton/Penguin, 2021) are a boxed set of postcards.

location. Alternatively, you might meet in the same place each week. Either way, you can draw on the richness of other-than-human nature around you, exploring the area to find the right place or materials that represent the transition. (See Chapter 10 for more information on how to work ethically and safely outdoors.)

Introducing the Intervention

Explain that you will ask the person to think about a particular transition and that there can be many components to a transition. These might include what we are transitioning from and to, things that are being let go of, uncertainty or fear about what is to come, the reasons why the transition is happening and our choices within it.

Explain that you are going to invite the person to represent their transition through nature and how you will do this. This might be choosing an image(s) from a selection, working with the image they have brought or finding something in the environment. Explain that they may choose to represent one or several components of the transition.

Explain that you will then ask them to talk you through the story of the transition they are representing, and that you will then ask some questions and explore the metaphor together further. As the therapist, you are not there to interpret, but to accompany the person in their own journey of making sense of their metaphor.

Check whether they have any questions and are happy to continue.

How to Facilitate the Technique

- Thinking about the transition you want to focus on, find an image or area that represents the transition.
- If relevant, lay out or display the images or items in a way that represents the transition (if using collage or collecting stones or objects from outdoors).
- "Briefly, tell me the story of your metaphor, image or creation."
- Clarify if the elements are all part of the same component in the transition or make up several components.
- Ask the person to say more about the different natural elements. This might include what they know and observe or the nature in their metaphor.

- Some examples might be:
  - "Tell me more about what the tides mean to you."
  - "What does the forked pathway mean?"
  - "I notice that the sky is cloudy today—does that mean anything to you?"
  - "I hear you mention the squirrels, could you say more about what they represent?"

The following questions are optional and may not all feel relevant. You may not have time to explore them all.

- If the landscape/plant/animal had a message, what would it say?
- Explore the relationship between the different elements.
- Some examples might be:
  - "How do the seagulls feel about the waves?"
  - "What would the stones say to the tide? What would the tide say in response?"
  - "You tell me how the bare branches feel now they have lost their leaves. Do the fallen leaves have any feelings or anything to say?"
- In other-than-human nature, there are often many opportunities for exploring letting go, making mistakes and choice (or lack of choice). These may arise within the metaphor—not wanting the tide to change, sadness or fear about the falling of leaves, growing through the cracks, fear of being hurt, being carried along by the tide or crowded out by a more dominant species.

If relevant, we might invite exploration of these themes using these questions:

- What does the pebble know about choice? How old does the pebble feel?
- What role have you given the grey squirrel? Does that say anything about the squirrel and the other elements that are significant for you?
- How might nature rectify a "mistake"?
- What are the risks of doing/not doing?
- What might this element of the transition/the transition as a whole look like if it was less managed and wilder?

- Finding meaning as we transition from a loss can be a helpful part of the transition. Is there anything in the metaphor/image that needs to change to have a big enough "why"? What needs to happen to make it more compelling?

This may be an opportunity to invite or offer further knowledge or observation of the plant/animal/landscape. For example, "I hear how stuck you feel as you describe the tree. I wonder how you'd feel if I were to share something about yew trees?" If they are happy for you to continue, "Yew tree branches grow downwards and when they reach the ground can root and form a new trunk. Is there anything that a natural process like this may change for you?"

Ending the Session

With sufficient time to close the session safely, let the person know you will be finishing soon. Ask them how they would like to leave their image/metaphor. They may want to take a collage home (make sure you have established whether or not this is possible at the beginning of the session) or throw pebbles or pinecones into the sea or trees. They might want to take a photo or quickly sketch an element to reflect on further or keep beyond the session. They may be happy to walk away.

How and When it Can Be Used

The exploration could be used for any life transition that someone wants to explore. It could be used for changes someone has chosen to move towards—moving house or deciding to end a relationship, for example. It may be particularly helpful for working with transitions that someone is thrown into and has no control over—living after a loved one has died, being made redundant, environmental degradation or a changing climate. Whether the transition is chosen or not, there can be a whole array of feelings and aspects to their experience that someone might find helpful to explore.

This technique could be used at different stages of loss and grief. It aims to bring a here-and-now perspective to illuminate, explore and understand how the person is experiencing their grief as a transition/change—from being with, to being without (or anticipating being without), to beyond. Different questions and invitations may be more appropriate at different points depending on where and how the person is in the transition. This is where your knowledge of and relationship with the person will help inform which questions you ask and whether you revisit the exploration another time with additional questions. For example, someone might be considering starting a new relationship after the death of a spouse. They might be questioning the decision and be pulled in many directions. Questions around letting go and exploring reasons for the change might be more relevant than questions around choice. On the other hand, if someone is angry and resentful, seeking unobtainable external closure or in denial about the death of someone or the end of a relationship, questions relating to choice and letting go may be most helpful.

Working with nature as co-therapist to help identify and convey how we feel inherently connects us with nature. Working sensitively with someone's existing relationship with nature in mind can be a way to foster and nurture a positive, secure attachment with an outdoor space, enabling the conditions for the actualising tendency, self-actualisation, psychological growth and healing. This can be particularly valuable if we need a safe space to grieve and perhaps do not have this with friends or family, or if our grief is disenfranchised (when how we feel is not accepted by society and/or family and friends, or even ourselves). Taking our grief into nature can be a way to be seen, heard and held in our experience.

Working with nature gives us the opportunity to invite in a wider perspective. This might be helpful if someone feels stuck and unable to see or feel anything other than the acuteness of loss, pain, fear or aloneness in a situation. Inviting in a metaphor that engages other life can help make space to explore the connection with other people, pursuits, feelings, hopes and roles if and when someone is able. In relation to the dual process model, this may be helpful if someone is or feels stuck in a loss-oriented process.

We can also work with nature to focus on an internal aspect of our experience, working with what we observe and know of other-than-human nature to bring in new ways of exploring our inner experience of the transition. This might involve taking a closer look at what is happening in the nature used to represent a particular aspect of the transition. Or it might involve thinking about what else is known about the other-than-human nature used. Perhaps a closed oyster shell represents how someone feels about beginning a new relationship after the death of a partner. They may see the layers of protection in the shell. Perhaps a vulnerable, broken heart is the pearl within.

The therapist may invite the person to share what else they know or observe about pearls and oysters, or may ask if they can share what else they themselves know or observe. This might be that oysters can change sex as they age, or that newly spawned oysters create their own shell by filtering calcium from the water, sometimes attaching to old oyster shells. Or it might be that there are many barnacles and other creatures living on the shell. This information and observation may not be significant for the person's metaphor and experience; and should always be offered and the person asked whether it means anything for them. It may open up an additional perspective or association, enabling a greater understanding or shift in the transition.

Sometimes, just seeing that our own experience is shared more widely (in human and/or other-than-human nature) can help us feel less alone and more trusting or accepting of our process. This in itself can be helpful in navigating transitions.

References/Attributions

ChrisLin Method by Christina Bachini and Lindsey Wheeler is licensed under Attribution 4.0 International. (Shorter, more common version: ChrisLin Method by Christina Bachini and Lindsey Wheeler is licensed under CC BY 4.0.)

ChrisLin Method and Technique Steps or Frameworks by Christina Bachini and Lindsey Wheeler is licensed under Attribution 4.0 International. (Shorter, more common version: ChrisLin Method and Technique Steps or Frameworks by Christina Bachini and Lindsey Wheeler is licensed under CC BY 4.0.)

Totten, N. (2011). *Wild Therapy: Undomesticating Inner and Outer Worlds*. Ross-on-Wye: PCCS Books.

CHAPTER 2

Doll Making and Traumatic Loss
From Rag Doll to Riches

Sharon Strouse

Historical Perspective

Dolls as unique objects are carved, shaped, bound and stitched into the fabric of our collective history from ancient to modern times. We share an inherent human need to create self-images for a variety of mystical, magical and practical purposes (Nikouei & Nasirabadi, 2016). Crafted from found materials such as wood, bone, clay, ivory, stone, leather, cloth and wax, they are carriers of cultural heritage and commonly included in prestigious museum collections around the world.

Some of the oldest known dolls are Japanese dogū dolls—earthen humanoid figures, 14,000–400 BC—and wooden paddle dolls discovered in Egyptian tombs—companions in the afterlife, 2000 BC. The Greeks and Romans deposited dolls in their temples, believing in their life-sustaining powers. Effigy dolls, used in rituals to cast spells, are well documented in African, Native American and European cultures where they evolved into the poppet dolls of folk magic. Akuba fertility dolls from Ghana are wooden disk-shaped figurines, carried by women hoping to have children. Native American Hopi kachina dolls, carved out of cottonwood root and hung on adobe walls, served to educate and remind the tribe of deceased ancestors who were believed to mediate between human and spirit worlds.

Although dolls were thought to have spiritual, magical and ritual value throughout the ancient world, they also served intrinsic human needs. Dolls as artifacts of comfort date back to the Bronze Age and a soapstone doll buried with a child. Rag dolls discovered in the graves of Roman children, 300 BC, as well as thousand-year-old corn husk dolls found across the maze-producing areas of the world, point to the doll as our most ancient toy (Young, 1992). They are prime examples of dolls created from bits and pieces of material such as stone, cloth and corn husks, and formed into human likeness. They are both self-symbols and symbols of something greater. "They teach and have power, they stimulate the imagination, and have the potential to speak and to provide companionship" (Feen-Calligan, McIntire & Sands-Goldstein, 2009, p.172).

Today, dolls and doll making hold significant value in the lives of both children and adults, regardless of gender. They serve a variety of purposes and are found in a wide range of settings from transitional plaything and treasured collectable to transformational objects in the treatment of complex trauma (Stance, 2014). They are valuable art therapy tools, not only in the process of making and shaping but as a means of expression through interaction and play (Vollmann, 1997, 2017). They are of benefit in assisted living facilities with dementia patients (Mitchell, McCormack & McCance, 2014), in hospital settings with children (Gaynard, Goldberg & Laidley, 1992), in cases of childhood sexual abuse (Klorer, 1995), in the processing of traumatic grief (Feen-Calligan *et al.*, 2009) and as vehicles for self-growth, development and discovery (Krystyniak, 2020).

Gossamer Impressions

My early experience of doll making with my mother comes to me in bits and pieces, less as memory and more as gossamer impressions held in my body. Warm sunlight filters through trees, and we sit on a blanket on the ground with old socks. My small hands move over heavy textured cotton—is it the toe or heel I hold? A large silver needle moves through a black buttonhole. I do not remember the face, but the smell of nail polish comes to me, and a small, tender mouth takes form. Strips are cut from a companion sock, rolled, stuffed and randomly top-stitched to become arms and legs. Is there brown yarn for hair? I am not sure, only sure of the glee and pride over my new rag doll. It is a very early memory, one that fades over the years but comes back into my consciousness and points me toward a healing.

Other than that single experience, I did not remember doll making during childhood or adolescence, and I did not make dolls with my two girls and son. I found it poignant when the notion to make a doll presented itself, so many years later, in the midst of a traumatic and complete unraveling. I was in the second year of bereavement, struggling in the aftermath of my 17-year-old daughter Kristin's suicide. My shattered identity and sense of purpose as a wife, mother, daughter, sister, friend and art therapist was redefined by way of mundane everyday tasks, including the issue of what to do with Kristin's things. I gave a lot of her clothes away, shipped them off to an orphanage in India, comforted in meeting a need. The rest hung in her closet, too precious, too saturated with memory to let go. On the day that doll making came to me, I stood in her room before opened closet doors. I was struck by the irony of it all: Kristin was to study fashion design in New York when she died. As I took in her smell, I wondered what it would be like to make a doll from the fabrics of her life. The idea drifted into my consciousness, and along with it, I remembered my mother and the sock doll we created. A thread connected my mother, me and my daughter across generations and over time and space. Yes, a doll—a perfectly terrifying idea under the circumstances.

I set a quiet time aside to make the selection and noticed my heightened anxiety as I ran my hands over her clothes. I settled on three shirts—a black velvet lace top, a gray cashmere sweater, and a white cotton tank. I could work with these and took the shirts into my basement art studio. This safe space contained me and invited my stillness as I created and felt myself again. There, I mercifully moved out of ordinary time into a creative meditative state (Strouse, 2013). I spent the early part of my grief journey playing with images torn from magazines, creating collages one after the other. I touched into the traumatic event of Kristin's suicide, in an effort to make sense of my life (Neimeyer, 2019). The art therapist in me was buried somewhere beneath the rubble, my private practice put aside as my attention turned inward. The fragments of my life safely arranged and rearranged themselves in a collage process of restorative retelling (Rynearson, 2001) that turned into a devotional practice. Creating was the only thing that assuaged the physical pain. I was a mother finding her way through the territory of unspeakable grief (Strouse, 2014).

I put paper scraps aside and took fabric into my hands. I began the process of creating a braided rag doll, to bring to life what lived in my imagination. I did not sit or stand at my art table but sat in the comfort of a softly padded barrel chair. I allowed my body a warm embrace as I took a first cut. My heart pounded, I was hot and sweaty. What if I made a mistake? I listened to my internal dialogue. "There are no mistakes, only opportunities. The worst thing already happened: she died." A swirl of autumn leaves outside the window caught my attention, reminding me that all of nature lets go.

I cut the three shirts into long strips and let them fall into a pile on the floor. That was all I could do that first day.

Over subsequent days, I braided and rebraided, black, gray and white together, and struggled with forming the doll's head, with forming the doll's body and attaching the arms and legs. In the end, shiny black eyes were sewn on, snippets of shirt fabric became hair, and a small red heart button was attached to the chest. My rag doll was long and lanky, soft and pliable. She sat with sad eyes and looked back at me.

Doll making served my powerful desire to reconnect with my child, an attempt to tightly weave together what was broken, and to nurture and protect what was beyond my grasp. It was a disquieting process; doing the work is sometimes like that. Years later, I understood this slow-paced mending, within the context of attachment-informed grief therapy (Kosminsky & Jordan, 2016), specifically the work of Klass, Silverman and Nickman (1996) which emphasized the importance of a continuing bond with the deceased. 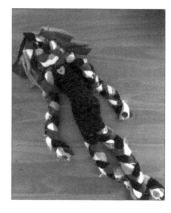 Satisfied with what I learned from the doll-making process, I delved back into what collage offered. I was in need of very deep dives into the razor-sharp edges of meaning reconstruction, an exploration of the event itself, her suicide and who I was now (Neimeyer, 2019). I put Kristin on a shelf in my studio, in a spot where she could keep an eye on me.

Survivors of Traumatic Loss

Over time, I returned to my professional life, my local art therapy private practice, and developed collage workshops for survivors and professionals at The Compassionate Friends (TCF), the American Foundation for Suicide Prevention (AFSP), the Association for Death Education and Counseling (ADEC) and the Tragedy Assistance Program for Survivors (TAPS) national conferences. It was within the context of my long-standing art therapy work with TAPS military suicide survivors that doll making came to mind with its specific therapeutic values of identity reformation and continuing bonds capacity (Krystyniak, 2020).

The Artful Grief: Open Art Studio was a fixture at the TAPS national conferences, available over the course of a three-day weekend. Since 2009, hundreds of survivors have entered the safe studio space that I founded and facilitated. It was well stocked and organized and offered a variety of art therapy modalities, such as collage, memory boxes, altered books, mask making, talking sticks, prayer flags and painted stones. The survivors' creative process and finished products served as agents of change (Moon, 2016). Each art therapy modality rested on the scaffolding of workshops and professional trainings as well as extensive personal experiences. We hold the space for our clients' healing experiences and must "cultivate a high capacity for distress tolerance—for remaining present in the face of emotional, cognitive, and behavioral storms" (Kosminsky & Jordan, 2016, p.123). With that comes personal knowledge of the territory in hand, and doll making was no exception.

Doll making served my powerful desire to reconnect with my child, an attempt to tightly weave together what was broken, and to nurture and protect what was beyond my grasp. It was a disquieting process, doing the work is sometimes like that.

I created nine dolls over several years, and each experience of cutting, stitching and mending taught me something new. The soft three-inch dolls taught me how simple wrapping and binding over a short period of time offers experiences of containment and soothing. Kristin's shiny palette knife became the head and hair of another doll, and I realized the powerful symbolic use of non-traditional objects in the creation of dolls. Long, lanky, bendable wire dolls offered experiences of control, pleasure in expression and posture. Larger 12-inch dolls invited intricate dressing with trim and lace, and a larger surface for the ever-present challenge of the doll's face, one I never fully mastered other than buttons or pins for eyes. Several doll bodies became sacred reliquaries. I placed Kristin's hair into a red satin heart and cross-stitched the applique shut. I placed a small stone, from the site where her body was found, into the open chest cavity of another doll, mended it closed, covered it with lace and attached a small silver heart. I experienced challenges and frustrations in the process of making and shaping as well as unexpected triumphs, all in service of a deep inner knowing that came not from the pages of a book but from the movement of my own body, my hands, as they touched all of it. In the process, I created tangible and long-lasting self-images as well as soft, pliable images of Kristin, which spoke of our continuing bond (Feen-Calligan *et al.*, 2009).

I was confident that my doll-making experience had prepared me for doll making at TAPS, which included the invitation to bring articles of clothing as well as their most precious possession—their loved one's military uniform. I knew what it was like to cut up clothing. I had cut up Kristin's shirts, dresses and beaded vests, but inviting the use of their military uniform felt different. The words "most precious" grabbed my attention, and my awareness went to the top shelf of Kristin's closet and settled on bunkalina, her tattered, torn baby blanket.

Transforming the Precious

I left bunkalina where it was for 17 years, undisturbed in the midst of the repetitive cleaning out and letting go. Bunkalina was a steady constant through the years, an untouchable sacred remnant. Bunkalina was a soft cotton baby blanket, given to Kristin when she was born, the one she chose over all others as her treasured companion, her comfort and object of love. She slept with it every night, up around her head and wrapped around the two middle fingers she sucked. When the pastel plaid friend faded and the middle part of the baby blanket disintegrated into tattered pieces, it was replaced by an exact replica, bunkalina two. Bunkalina two made it through middle school and through high school. We teased Kristin about taking it to college and bringing it with her on her honeymoon. We buried her with bunkalina two, while bunkalina one sat on the shelf, the last thread that connected me to her and her infancy.

I took bunkalina from Kristin's closet and brought it into the studio. It sat there for a few weeks. I allowed the idea of deconstructing and reconstructing the remnants to live in me for a while. I remember the day vividly; I wondered what it would be like and thought of doll making with my mother and the first braided doll I made. I stood at the table and held the torn pieces. They hung in gentle folds, and I wanted to capture that soft, unstructured look. I gathered my resolve and pulled the batting apart and made cuts in what was left of the fabric. The experience was surprisingly joyful. My attachment to the form of her blanket and its associated memories dissolved with a sense of relief. My attachments were heavy, imbedded in an old form, and they gave way to a softer and lighter relationship with the fabric and what it represented. I searched for a new form and was reminded of Levine's (2014) invitation to go beyond the normal everyday considerations and engage the world of imagination. That sweet moment sat side by side with the disquieting moment of the braided doll—joy, sorrow, life, death all woven together during a transformational process.

The Ghillie Suit Doll: Case Study

On a weekend in October, TAPS suicide survivors interested in doll making entered the studio and selected a soft, pliable muslin doll form in one of four sizes—three, five, eight or 12 inch. Fabrics, lace, trim, yarn, buttons, a variety of sewing materials and glue guns were provided. They could create a doll of their choosing, one that commemorated a lost love or one symbolic of themselves. They brought personal fabrics—articles of clothing, their loved one's military uniform—and cut and tore them into lasting, loving and tangible objects. They gathered at round tables for eight, facilitated by a team of skilled trauma-informed art therapists, and created together. There was a palpable energy in the room, an atmosphere penetrated by willingness, curiosity, courage and presence.

She caught my eye right away; I will call her Beverly to ensure confidentiality. She has given her full permission to share the compelling details of her experience. She was visually shaking, deeply traumatized by her son's suicide and unsure of what she wanted to create. Survivors suffering traumatic loss often experience feelings of shock, confusion, helplessness, rage, guilt and diminished self-worth, especially in such cases of suicide, homicide and accidental and untimely death (Kosminsky & Jordan, 2016). Beverly was immediately supported by one of the art therapists, as she walked around the studio considering the possibilities. She stopped at the table full of fabrics and picked up a bolt of brown burlap and soft flannel camouflage, and with a sense of purpose said, "I want to make a doll." The materials themselves were triggers to act, pointing to the critical importance of an abundant, well-stocked studio. Variety offers opportunity, simple choices empower and the sense of self is reinforced in the process (Strouse, Haas-Cohen & Bokoch, 2021).

Beverly joined an already robust table and quietly began to create. She cut camouflage material into pieces, slowly stitched it to the eight-inch doll's body and separated and pulled out long fibers of burlap into individual strips.

She knew how to sew—her mother taught her—and she settled into a slow, gentle rhythm which helped to soothe and comfort her. She covered her son's head with camouflage material and created a black mask over his mouth, leaving his piercing blue eyes visible. She attached long threads of burlap to all sides of her son's uniform and tucked white angel wings tightly beneath his body. Here we see properties of a meaning-making process come alive— bracing, pacing and facing (Neimeyer, 2019). Beverly experienced bracing, or support, when she entered the safe, non-judgmental studio and established a warm connection with the staff and survivors' community. She paced herself, slowly collected materials, slowly stitched, pulled out the burlap threads and eased into her story. She then faced the hardest parts, the details, where emotions rose and fell during an unfolding process of meaning reconstruction, "a process of reaffirming or reconstructing a world of meaning that has been challenged by loss" (Thompson & Neimeyer, 2014, p.4).

> My son was in Iraq, deployed as a sniper. He was excellent at what he did and saved many lives. He wore a ghillie suit, which he created with long pieces of burlap. It disguised him during dangerous missions. While troops were securing a terrorist stronghold, the entranceway to a home was blown open, killing a baby that was held in his mother's arms. My son then shot the mother in self-defense, before she shot him and the troops who were with him. In the aftermath of that horrific event, my son placed the baby back into the mother's arms, in a final act of compassion. The ravages of war offer up cruel and unusual punishments on all fronts, and he was subsequently bullied by his unit, called a "baby killer." Months later, he took his own life.

The Military was not forthcoming with the cause of his death, which added to the trauma of his loss. Rage.

This story was told countless times during the day—new pieces added, new memories woven in—as various survivors sat down at the table or bystanders inquired about the ghillie suit doll and its back story. Her first tellings were haunting, punctuated by anxious pauses and in some ways disconnected from those listening. That shifted over time. In her retelling, she placed herself into the narrative, as an engaged participant rather than horrified victim, which is central to restorative retelling (Rynearson, 2001), and important in the treatment of traumatic loss. She became more and more present to the story and aware of herself and what came to her during her tactile experience with the burlap ghillie suit. "My son crafted his own ghillie suit while he was still in the States. We often facetimed while he was sewing. He showed me how he pulled the long burlap threads, knotted and sewed them to his combat uniform. As I attached each thread to my doll, I remembered and felt my son's presence. We were creating together. I felt our bond getting stronger and stronger. I felt at peace for the very first time. My madness, worry and anger fell away." She also seemed to understand something of his struggle with depression. "The burlap was rough to the touch, it was hot and heavy, almost a burden...it was a protection that in the end destroyed him." The art therapist supported her, helped her make connections between the fabric's tactile experience and her story, which allowed her to come to terms with his suicide. "Working through traumatic material involves telling the story, making meaning, and re-authorship—retelling the story in a new way that expands upon the previous telling" (White & Epston, 1999, p.13).

At the day's end, Beverly was asked, "What does your son need now?" Unsure, a "wrapping" was suggested, which lit up her eyes. She assuaged her unyielding yearning for her son, satisfied her biological needs to nurture and protect, and brought closure to her intense experience. "I swaddled him, just like I did when he was a baby. He is both soldier and baby, in my arms." This specific directive served to contain, calm and soothe the mother and gave form to the retelling of her son's life and death.

The next day, Beverly came back to the art studio and was guided toward making a self-image doll. She dressed herself in black and white, a puritanical mantle that bespoke of guilt, shame and societal judgments embedded in the fabric of suicide loss. She appears stiff and rigid, in an attempt to guard and control her feelings. Slow, gentle, rhythmic sewing actions joined with aggressive cutting, stabbing and piercing motions. The qualities of these movements served to release powerful, aggressive emotions (Moon, 2014), 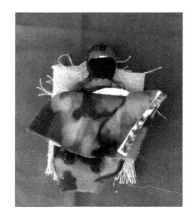 often a part of a suicide survivor's conscious and unconscious experiences. All were in service to healing.

Coincidentally, she used fabric that I donated to the TAPS studio—white lace from Kristin's pillowcase—which formed the white apron on Beverly's self-image doll. She unknowingly connected us and our traumatic loss, which was indeed magical. This was something I shared with her much later in her processing. Beverly went on to say, "I am a simple mother, my children are my life. My mouth is straight and closed shut, it is hard to talk about feelings, I cannot say much." She wears her son's dog tags and a necklace with his name, holds a burlap bag of expressed hopes and wishes, and looks at us with piercing blue eyes, as does her son. During the creation of her self-image doll, Beverly placed her ghillie-suit-clad son on the table, weaving him into her experience of self. Upon completion, she placed them together, arm in arm, mirroring her son's last compassionate act toward the deceased mother and baby in Iraq. "My heart is pounding, I am excited. I have love back, I feel love again, we are together." Only when there is a real sense of rawness and authentic connection to a more genuine sense of self can the beginning of a new, more adaptable one emerge (Van Lith, 2020). Beverly carried the two dolls with her during the remainder of the conference, either in her arms or sticking out of her purse, with countless additional opportunities to retell her story. "Dolls function ritually for protection, symbolic substitutions, and healings as well as, in everyday, as companions, symbols of attachment, and tools for communication" (Potash & Ho, 2014, p.29).

We had the pleasure of seeing Beverly a year later when she came back to the TAPS suicide survivors conference and shared how doll making was a significant transformative experience. She looked markedly different: more grounded, present, calmer and released from the severe trauma symptomology that plagued her during our prior meeting. "I took my dolls home and brought them to my psychiatrist, shared my doll-making experience, asked him to hold them, told him that talk therapy had not positively affected me like doll making had." Beverly placed her dolls 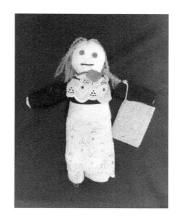 prominently in her china cabinet where she saw them together daily. "They are tangible reminders of my journey, my continued bond with my son, and my own evolution as a survivor and Gold Star mom."

Rag Doll to Riches

My own personal experience with doll making, which began with my rag doll, laid the groundwork for my work with survivors of traumatic loss at TAPS. I had a deep inner knowing of the creative process and could hold that space for others with compassion. I sensed a timeless quality in the restorative and assertive act of doll making, for myself and for Beverly. We were part of an ancient tradition that reached beyond time and space, connecting us to our mothers and to our deceased children. Our creative process and finished products served to integrate opposing forces within us and brought a sense of wholeness and fulfillment (Levine, 1992, p.77). Precious, personal fabrics were fertile grounds for our safe descents into the underworld of loss. I was confident that one's positive core strength would triumph (Strouse, 2020). Imagination pushed open the door of possibility during this non-verbal process with three-dimensional pliable human forms and offered us a glimpse of our future. Our self-image dolls were tangible reminders that post-traumatic growth is possible and contributed to our ongoing process of meaning reconstruction. Beverly and I gained a measure of self-control amidst the chaos of traumatic loss as we braided, stitched and mended, and retold our stories over time. These slow, repetitive self-soothing motions fulfilled our biological needs for care and protection and strengthened our continuing bonds with our children.

As Beverly left the Artful Grief studio with her two dolls, I glanced at my bunkalina doll on display, nestled against the wall. They were examples of transcendence. Love and loss were bound together in the tangible bodies of our dolls that rested in our arms and hearts.

Key Points

- Humans share a need to create self-images for mystical, magical and practical purposes.
- Dolls and doll making hold value for children and adults, regardless of gender.
- Doll making is a valuable art therapy tool, found in a wide range of clinical settings.
- Personal knowledge of the creative process is a clinician's ethical responsibility.

- Art materials are triggers to act and point to the importance of quality and abundance.
- A warm, non-judgmental, safe space supports bracing, pacing and facing.
- Doll making supports a continuing bond with the deceased and meaning reconstruction.
- The creative process and tactile experience with fabrics supports restorative retelling.
- Doll making satisfies a biological need to nurture and protect our offspring.
- A self-image doll is a tangible reminder of transformation.

References

Feen-Calligan, H., McIntire, B. & Sands-Goldstein, M. (2009). Art therapy applications of dolls in grief recovery, identity, and community service. *Art Therapy: Journal of the American Art Therapy Association, 26*(4), 167–173.

Gaynard, L., Goldberger, J. & Laidley, L.N. (1992). The use of stuffed, body outline dolls with hospitalized children and adolescents. *Child Health Care, 20*(4), 216–224.

Klass, D., Silverman, P.R. & Nickman, S.L. (1996). *Continuing Bonds: New Understandings of Grief*. New York, NY: Routledge.

Klorer, G. (1995). Use of anatomical dolls in play and art therapy with sexually abused children. *The Art is Psychotherapy, 22*(5), 467–473.

Kosminsky, P.S. & Jordan, J.R. (2016). *Attachment-Informed Grief Therapy: The Clinician's Guide to Foundations and Applications*. New York, NY: Routledge.

Krystyniak, J. (2020). The Use of Dolls and Figures in Therapy: A Literature Review. *Expressive Therapies Capstone Theses*, 321. https://digitalcommons.lesley.edu/expressive_theses/321

Levine, S.K. (1992). *Poiesis: The Language of Psychology and the Speech of the Soul*. Toronto: Palmerston Press.

Levine, S.K. (2014). Poiesis, Praise and Lament: Celebration, Mourning and the "Architecture" of Expressive Arts Therapy. In B.E. Thompson & R.A. Neimeyer (eds) *Grief and the Expressive Arts: Practices for Creating Meaning*. New York, NY: Routledge.

Mitchell, G., McCormack, B. & McCance, T. (2014). Therapeutic use of dolls for people living with dementia: A critical review of the literature. *Dementia, 15*(5), 976–1001. https://doi.org/10.1177/1471301214548522

Moon, B.L. (2016). *Art-Based Group Therapy: Theory and Practice*. Springfield, IL: Charles C. Thomas.

Moon, C.H. (2014). *Materials and Media in Art Therapy: Critical Understandings of Diverse Artistic Vocabularies*. New York, NY: Routledge.

Neimeyer, R.A. (2019). Meaning reconstruction in bereavement: Development of a research program. *Death Studies, 43*(2), 79–81. https://doi.org/10.1080/07481187.2018.1456620

Nikouei, A. & Nasirabadi, M.S. (2016). Study of the importance of contemporary Iranian traditional handmade dolls and puppets. *Wacana Seni Journal of Arts Discourse, 15*, 27–61. http://dx.doi.org/10.21315/ws2016.15.2

Potash, J.S. & Ho, R.T.H. (2014). Expressive Therapies for Bereavement: The State of the Arts. In B.E. Thompson & R.A. Neimeyer (eds) *Grief and the Expressive Arts: Practices for Creating Meaning*. New York, NY: Routledge.

Rynearson, E.K. (2001). *Retelling Violent Death*. New York, NY: Routledge.

Stance, S.M. (2014). Therapeutic doll making in art psychotherapy for complex trauma. *Art Therapy: Journal of the American Art Therapy Association, 31*(1), 12–20. https://doi.org/10.1080/07421656.2014.873689

Strouse, S.T. (2013). *Artful Grief: A Diary of Healing*. Bloomington, IN: Balboa Press.

Strouse, S.T. (2014). Collage: Integrating the Torn Pieces. In B.E. Thompson & R.A. Neimeyer (eds) *Grief and the Expressive Arts: Practices for Creating Meaning*. New York, NY: Routledge.

Strouse, S.T. (2020). Artful grief: An art therapy application of appreciative living. *AI Practitioner, 22*(2), 5–12.

Strouse, S., Haas-Cohen, N., & Bokoch, R. (2021). Benefits of an open art studio to military suicide survivors. *The Arts in Psychotherapy, 72*(1), 101722. https://doi.org/10.1016/j.aip.2020.101722

Thompson, B.E. & Neimeyer, R.A. (2014). *Grief and the Expressive Arts: Practices for Creating Meaning*. New York, NY: Routledge.

Van Lith, T. (2020). Fostering client voice and choice through art therapy. *Art Therapy: Journal of the American Art Therapy Association, 37*(4), 167–168.

Vollmann, S. (1997). Doll making and play: A therapeutic modality for an adolescent boy with gender identity disorder. *Pratt Institute Creative Arts Therapy Review, 18*, 76–86.

Vollmann, S. (2017). Multimedia Approaches in Childhood Bereavement. In B. MacWilliam (ed.) *Complicated Grief, Attachment, & Art Therapy: Theory, Treatment, and 14 Ready-to-Use Protocols*. London and Philadelphia, PA: Jessica Kingsley Publishers.

White, M. & Epston, D. (1999). *Narrative Means to Therapeutic Ends*. New York, NY: W.W. Norton & Company.

Young, R. (1992). *Dolls*. New York, NY: Dillon Press.

CHAPTER 3

Memory Boxes

Containers of Love and Loss
Sarah Vollmann

Ellen, a grieving mom who lost her daughter to suicide, sat with me in the art therapy studio. She pulled a ziplock bag from her purse that held small scraps of her daughter's clothing, and explained that she had commissioned someone to make her a quilt; these fabric remnants were the leftover pieces. She gently took them out of the bag, smoothing them with her hands. There were shirt cuffs, strips of lace trim, T-shirt hems, and pockets from her daughter's military uniform. She quietly said that they were too precious to throw away, but that she did not know what to do with them. As we looked at the remnants together, we discussed their poignant symbolization of her grieving process. The questions raised were important. What does one do, after a traumatic loss, with the pieces that are left behind? Is there a way to integrate them, to hold them, and to somehow find meaning?

I offered Ellen the possibility of creating a memory box, and she expressed immediate interest. Various sizes and shapes of boxes were available, and she selected a rectangular box made of sturdy cardboard. To begin, she decided to write a letter to her daughter, which she carefully folded and enclosed in the box. She then glued the box shut, in an act that was reminiscent of a burial. The letter was safely, privately, and permanently encased. Finally, she lovingly wrapped the box with the fragments of her daughter's clothing, covering all surfaces of the box and using a glue gun to adhere the fabric. Pockets became holders for mementos. A small watercolor painting of a blue heart, representing love and sorrow, was visibly placed in one pocket. She collaged her daughter's name around the heart and added an image of the moon to represent her daughter's beloved zodiac sign. Remaining strips of lace and shirt cuffs, with buttons still attached, were draped from other pockets, so that all fabric remnants found their place and were included. Silver charms were tucked inside pockets as symbols of love. She embellished a piece of the army uniform with the words "army" and "fierce," and said that her daughter's military experience was a vital part of her identity. A decal of a butterfly in flight was added to represent her daughter's departure, and her loss. She hugged the box to her chest after reflecting upon its significance and told me that she would keep it on her mantle. It had become a transformative memorial object, important in its process and as a final product.

Art therapists often offer boxes as an expressive modality for grieving patients. In a creative arts therapy context, boxes can organically encourage exploration, expression, and healing, and they connect to traditions and rituals from across history and cultures. Museums around the world display boxes as beloved and common artifacts. In New York's Metropolitan Museum of Art, boxes are abundantly dispersed throughout many collections. An Egyptian Shabti box of gessoed wood is delicately painted, with slender stripes of green, blue, and deep red. It was created with a funerary purpose in approximately 1250 BC and was placed inside a tomb. Painted wood figurines known as shabti figures were contained inside and were meant to carry out manual labor in the afterlife on behalf of the deceased. A lacquer box from the 12th century hails from Korea. It is adorned with chrysanthemums in inlaid mother-of-pearl and served as a container for incense in tea ceremonies. A rectangular American box from 1675 is carved of oak and pine, chiseled with geometric flowers and leaves. It has a hinged lid and served as the holder of valuables and important documents. A square German writing box from approximately 1715 is made of oak, cedar, exotic hardwood, ebonized fruitwood, and silver, with marquetry in pewter, brass, and tortoiseshell. A luxurious object that contained writing and sealing implements, its elaborate design and preciousness were a reflection of its owner's aristocratic status, and it had a ceremonial purpose in the court. A wooden treasure box was carved by the Māori people of Aotearoa, also known as New Zealand, in 1850. It contains four feathers. Designed to hold personal ornaments, Māori treasure boxes hold feathers or pendants which become imbued with the supernatural powers of their wearer after contact occurs. Māori treasure boxes were hung in the rafters of a house to safeguard their holdings. A Russian spice box from 1900 resembles a miniature tower with a spire and is crafted in silver. It was utilized in a Jewish ritual that marks the end of the holy Sabbath, in which a candle and spice essence were used as a blessing. Each box is distinct, with valued ceremonial and personal significance, and the collective illuminates their timeless and worldwide appeal.

The universality and therapeutic relevance of boxes can be explained by their unique qualities and functions. They evoke varied associations and responses due to their diverse appearances and the range of materials that are used to create and embellish them. Boxes may be viewed as symbols of self, with an inside and an outside. As containers, they can enclose items of our choosing, and in a therapy context, they offer a potential receptacle for all feelings, including frightening, confusing, contradictory, or painful material. Kaufman (1996, p.237) reminds us that the definition of contain, "to hold within fixed limits; to enclose; to hold," and its synonyms, "to retain, have, keep, comprehend, embrace, and embody," evoke the holding space between therapist and patient, as described by Devine (1994, p.99) as "free and protected space" in which profound work may occur. Weller (2015, p.147) elaborates that:

> all deep work requires a holding space, a secure vessel within which the work is carried out. Vessels both contain and separate, allowing us to attend to the matter at hand. The container must be constructed slowly, however, over time, with attention, repetition, and care.

As we consider the importance of containment in any therapy process, we can appreciate the power of introducing a palpable box as a creative object to augment treatment. Kaufman (1996) explains that various forms of containers often productively coexist in art therapy treatment like Russian nesting dolls, including the patient–therapist relationship, the process of art making, as "art is a container for feelings and a means of expressing them" (p.242), art therapy itself, where "the infinity of the unconscious is accessed" (p.246), and, if implemented, the art therapy box, which can safely hold overwhelming or unspeakable content. The box's lid may be closed as needed, to secure or guard its contents and to promote regulation, mastery, safety, and control. The limiting context of a box and its restricted space provides distance for the client and can make issues feel more manageable (Farrell-Kirk, 2001). Art therapy boxes furnish a tangible safe space that may be touched, manipulated, repeatedly reworked, and transformed.

As boxes have an outside and an inside, they can easily obscure their holdings, providing intimacy and secrecy. Kaufman (1996, p.237) describes a box's "secret magic space with immensity and intimacy... A complete and private world." It is impossible to see all sides of a box at once. They are multifaceted, and the union of their panels and facets provides a model of integration (Farrell-Kirk, 2001). Their functions are assorted and sometimes contradictory; they can unveil and protect, expose or hide. Boxes can guard their contents from the viewer, or they can shield the viewer from contents that are too difficult to face. Their marked presence in art history adds to their sense of value, which is reinforced by their frequent purpose as jewelry boxes, treasure chests, and the holders of precious items. I agree with Farrell-Kirk (2001, p.89), who explains:

> placing something in a box can not only signify the inherent value of the thing, but can actually imbue a mundane object with newfound importance... This connotation of value makes the box an effective tool in art therapy because it enables clients to signify the importance of the symbols or items placed within it.

When items are chosen, set apart, and placed into a box, they enter a three-dimensional frame that automatically conveys their shifted status into a world of symbol and cherished significance.

Sacred items are frequently contained in boxes, including the remains of the dead. Some boxes, like Egyptian sarcophagi, served as elaborate coffins. They were ornamented to honor the deceased and to fulfill mortuary traditions, and contained mummified remains. Eyes were traditionally depicted on the exterior to give the deceased an ongoing view of the world, and the name of the deceased was inscribed to ensure a transition into the afterlife. The stone sarcophagi of Ancient Rome served a similar function. Most were decoratively chiseled on the exterior with imagery to document the life of the deceased. In both cultures, the sarcophagi provided a hallowed holder for the body of the deceased while also enabling rituals pertaining to loss and remembrance. Farrell-Kirk (2001) explains that sarcophagi unite time; they were created in the present, memorialize the past by holding remains of the deceased, and impart a legacy into the future.

Reliquaries are another example of historic boxes created to hold our most revered contents. They were designed to contain the relics of a saint and traditionally held a piece of a saint's physical remains or a fragment of their clothing. Due to their hallowed contents, they are usually ornate and made from the most prized materials, including rare gemstones and precious metals. Some were created to resemble the body part that they contain, such as arm or feet reliquaries. New York City's Metropolitan Museum of Art has many reliquaries in its collection. A silver, casket-shaped reliquary from 1173 contains a relic of an English saint, Thomas Becket. The story of his life is etched in niello onto the box's panels. A French reliquary from approximately 1220 is sculpted as a bust of St. Yrieix, and once contained his skull. It is made of silver, rock crystal, and glass, and was carried in processions on feast days. A Swiss reliquary from the 14th century is shaped to represent the arm of St. Valentine. Made of silver, gilt, and sapphire, it was used in public processions and displayed upon the church altar for worship. The hand is sculpted in a gesture of blessing. The juxtaposition of an opulent and decorative reliquary that holds a human skull or toe is striking; it illustrates a box's capacity to be highly beautiful while also containing an item that some might consider to be morbid or grotesque. Polarities can often seamlessly coexist within the structure of a box, promoting integration in a therapeutic context. Like reliquaries, memory boxes can symbolize and evoke varied affect states and experiences, including grief and love.

Boxes used for remembrance customarily assist with meaning making, which is a prevalent need for the bereaved. Neimeyer (2012) states that a significant loss causes disruption to our life narrative. Attig (1996) explains that we often have to relearn the self and relearn the world after loss, because our worldview and identity are shaken. As we grieve, we often strive to make sense of our loss through rebuilding a life narrative that preserves continuity with who we were, before the death, while also integrating the reality of our changed worldview and sense of self (Neimeyer, Prigerson & Davies, 2002). In his theory of meaning reconstruction, Neimeyer (2012) describes the therapeutic value of processing both the event story, to make sense of the death, and the backstory of the relationship to the deceased, to address unfinished business and foster a continuing bond. He also describes a process of restorative retelling, based on the work of Rynearson (2001), in which the sharing and evolution of our narratives after loss assist with healing and growth. There are three steps that Neimeyer identifies in the restorative re-telling process. First, we brace ourselves to prepare for the therapeutic work, building readiness and a sense of safety. We then pace ourselves, easing into the exploration and sharing of difficult content while honoring our needs for time, defenses, and protection. Finally, as we feel able and ready, we face the story and our feelings, sharing about it in an in-depth way and beginning the process of integrating it into our life narrative.

Art therapy memory boxes can fluidly enable the process of meaning reconstruction, as illustrated in the following case study. In her memory box process, Kate, a bereaved adolescent who lost her mother, uses imagery, the art-making process, and the safe container provided by the box and the therapy relationship to explore her mother's illness, their relationship, and her intense grief. Bracing, pacing, and facing occurred, as frightening and overwhelming feelings that had not yet been explored were contained and gradually given voice. Unconscious content was given form, and the integration of her varied feelings and experiences, held together in the box, encouraged her own process of integrating the loss into her identity and life story.

My work with Kate, a teenage girl, began a few months after her mother died of an illness. Her family was very private about their loss because of their cultural background. Kate did not tell a single friend that her mother died, and her school was not informed. She was referred to me after her father incidentally disclosed the loss to a teacher during a conversation about her academics. She and her father seemed glad to access therapeutic support and she willingly engaged in weekly sessions. Kate soon revealed that her mom was her closest caregiver and favorite person.

Early in our work together, I suggested the possibility of creating a memory box. Kate enthusiastically selected a rectangular wooden box with a clasp. She wanted to paint it pink, as that was her mom's favorite color, and she carefully mixed colors to get the perfect hue. After experimenting with paintbrushes, she chose a smooth one that left minimal brush marks, and began painting the box's exterior with even strokes. I was surprised to see her paint over the clasp and hinges. She seemed to want to cover every surface in an even blanket of pink. I gently cautioned that painting over a closed box's hinges, edges, and clasp could permanently seal it shut, but reinforced that she could proceed as she wished. She nodded her understanding and explained that it was important to paint all surfaces.

In our next session, we inspected the box and discovered that it was painted shut. The box looked pristine and untouched as it had no visible brush strokes, and it was firmly sealed and covered in paint. It seemed like a perfect symbolization of Kate's experience of keeping her loss contained, hidden, and unaccessed, and of her hesitancy to look within. After several unsuccessful attempts to pry the box open, Kate proposed bringing it home to seek her father's help. I sensed a deep significance in her choice to reach out to her father for assistance, as it provided a means to share her mourning and memorialization, to build closeness, and to seek her dad's support for her engagement in therapy.

She arrived at her following session with a smile. Her father had successfully opened the box without scratching it. His support seemed to make it more feasible for her to delve into the creation of a memorial object, and to explore some of her repressed and unspoken feelings. She selected an image with large red dots to collage onto the top of the box. While she was not conscious of it at the time, she later realized that the image reflected symptoms of her mother's illness. She created a frame around it of pink fabric flower petals and shared about the pink flowers that they had recently placed on her mother's grave. She glued metallic hearts on all corners of the box, making everything very symmetrical and seeming to seek control and order in that process.

With clay, Kate molded small orbs that she colored pink and glued around the bottom perimeter of the box. They were extremely fragile and seemed to represent Kate's vulnerability. I wondered aloud if they would break if left unprotected. As a creative solution she added a sturdy panel of wood beneath them, and promptly painted it pink. It elevated the box and provided protection and a solid base, like a small altar.

The box's secure grounding seemed to encourage Kate's capacity to look within. Kate selected two photographs of guinea pigs for the inside of her box, one large and one small, which she placed together to represent herself and her mom. Inside the box's lid, she adhered an image of vibrant vegetables that were infused with light, using food as an apt symbol for the nurturance that her mother had provided. In this box, the guinea pigs clearly had all that they needed. Sadness emanated from her during this process. She used a copious amount of pink sequins to frame the vegetable image. Like her flower-petal frame, it provided an additional container for her strong feelings and symbolized her attempts to hold things together. The shimmer of the sequins also seemingly served as a defense, brightening a box that held sad and bleak feelings.

To finish, she glued a dark image with tree-like branches on the outer back of the box, in a spot that was barely visible. Unlike the rest of the box, it was asymmetrical and glued at a crooked angle, and its darkness contrasted with the cheerful pink background. Its juxtaposition seemed to give voice to her underlying feelings, which were not orderly or bright, and were present but mostly kept out of sight. She eventually concluded that the motion of the branches symbolized a sense of reaching and longing.

Kate's memory box was a heartfelt memorial for her mom and an integral vehicle of her treatment process. The restorative retelling concepts of bracing, pacing, and facing as described by Neimeyer (2016) were shown both in her creative process and in her finished art piece. She braced herself as she gathered art supplies with care, preparing herself for the unfolding that would occur while creating a memorial object. She then paced herself, using the fluid nature of the paint to self-soothe, and taking time to problem-solve when contending with a sealed box. Finally, she faced some of the intensity of her grief and experience, cracking open a box that had been tightly shut and placing images inside to symbolize love, longing, and the depth of her connection to her mom. The box's seamless color and symmetry gave Kate a needed sense of control. Unconscious fears and questions about her mom's illness and the death story were given form in an image that evoked her mother's journey. The depth of her grief was illustrated in a dark branch-like image that expressed underlying feelings that were difficult to tolerate. The integration of polarities was fostered, as the somber and slanted image, which sharply contrasted with the box's orderly and bright pink exterior, was given space within the box's facets and could be seen or hidden depending upon the angle of the viewer. The box's pink flower border echoed the solemn and hallowed space of her mother's grave, and its pristine, altar-like qualities visually affirmed its purpose as a commemorative object.

Kate's box also served the purpose of furthering a continuing bond to her mom. Klass, Silverman, and Nickman (1996) explain that the bereaved often maintain an important, ongoing connection to the deceased despite their physical absence, and that preserving a continuing bond to a lost loved one can be healthy, comforting, and adaptive. Art therapy memory boxes can tangibly assist in marking, preserving, and memorializing enduring relationships to lost loved ones. Kate decided to keep her box on her bedside table. She placed cherished mementos of her mother inside, including photos, a valentine, and a necklace that was one of her mom's last gifts for her. She said that she often looked at it before falling asleep or when she awoke in the morning, and that it was comforting, as it kept her mother close.

Art therapy memory boxes are as individual as their makers, as they are intricately personalized. The bereaved can imaginatively create and utilize their boxes as they see fit, and tailor them to best meet their needs. Like Kate, Ellen used her box to foster meaning reconstruction, but her process unfolded with its own unique and needed trajectory. Ellen's act of writing her last words to her daughter, and of containing and putting those words to rest, provided a self-described sense of peace and relief. While she chose to keep the contents of her letter private, it seemed to assist her in addressing the backstory of their relationship and some unfinished business. Her rehoming of unmoored and cherished remnants of her daughter's clothing into her art piece allowed her to begin a process of integration, reconstructing meaning as fragments were transformed into something new and whole. Her box also fostered a continuing bond, becoming a treasured keepsake that was prominently displayed to honor and remember her daughter. She expressed feelings of solace at having pieces of her daughter's clothing readily accessible and at her fingertips, to touch, connect, and remember.

As memorial objects, art therapy memory boxes can contain contradictory, unconscious, and painful material, including grief and love. In creating them, their makers may uncover new insights, tend to a continuing bond, rework their attachment relationship to the deceased, and reconfigure a disrupted life narrative. Boxes can hold our most precious, secret, painful, or vulnerable pieces, unveiling and protecting, allowing for exploration and refuge. Their contents can be expanded or altered over time, and their maker can choose to share or obscure what is kept inside. As we seal or open our memory boxes, we enter realms of ritual and transformation, reshaping our narrative of love and loss.

References

Attig, T. (1996). *How We Grieve: Relearning the World*. New York, NY: Oxford University Press.

Devine, L. (1994). The free and protected space: A mirror of the alchemical process. *Journal of Sandplay Therapy*, *3*(2), 97–104.

Farrell-Kirk, R. (2001). Secrets, symbols, synthesis, and safety: The role of boxes in art therapy. *Art Therapy: Journal of the American Art Therapy Association*, *39*(3), 88–92.

Kaufman, A.B. (1996). Art in boxes: An exploration of meanings. *The Arts in Psychotherapy*, *23*(3), 237–247.

Klass, D., Silverman, P.R. & Nickman, S.L. (1996). *Continuing Bonds: New Understandings of Grief*. New York, NY: Routledge.

Neimeyer, R.A. (ed.) (2012). *Techniques of Grief Therapy: Creative Practices for Counseling the Bereaved*. New York, NY: Routledge.

Neimeyer, R.A. (2016). Meaning reconstruction in the wake of loss: Evolution of a research program. *Behaviour Change*, *33*(2), 65–79.

Neimeyer, R.A, Prigerson, H.G. & Davies, B. (2002). Mourning and meaning. *American Behavioral Scientist*, *46*(2), 235–251.

Rynearson, E.K. (2001). *Retelling Violent Death*. New York, NY: Routledge.

Weller, F. (2015). *The Wild Edge of Sorrow: Rituals of Renewal and the Sacred Work of Grief*. Berkeley, CA: North Atlantic Books.

CHAPTER 4

Music as Companion and Consolation

Catharine DeLong

There was a moment in time when my life as I knew it fell apart—when loss was the air I breathed. Within a six-month period, my marriage of 27 years came to an end; I moved out of my home and across the country, leaving friends and my work as a freelance harpist; I parted ways with organized religion; and a beloved friend died unexpectedly. It was a time of being completely undone and unmoored, so I leaned into the one thing I knew. I sat down at my harp, the instrument I played since the age of 11, as a creative way to be with my grief, and I made music to tend to the ache in my heart (Schroeder-Sheker, 2001).

A Music Thanatology Journey

A few years prior to this avalanche of grief, I had watched Ted Koppel's *Nightline* interview featuring Therese Schroeder-Sheker (Schroeder-Sheker, 2001), the founder of music thanatology in the 1970s. It was December 25, 1996. There was something about serving a marginalized community of dying individuals that resonated with me. I reflected on that interview while getting my feet under me, with awareness that I was comforting myself during a liminal time by making music. This was self-care—a compassionate way to be with my sadness and to focus my energy during a traumatic time of loss. Perhaps I could also use my music skills to tend to the physical and spiritual needs of people nearing the end of life. And so it began.

The first thing I learned in music thanatology school was the principle of *cymatics*, a term deriving from Greek, meaning "wave form," used to describe the way that sound organizes matter (Jenny, 2001). The next lesson was related to the word thanatology itself. Derived from the name *Thanatos*, the god of death in Greek mythology, thanatology refers to the study of death and dying.

Music thanatology takes inspiration from the Benedictine monks of 11th-century Cluny, France, who cultivated an awareness that music comforts body, mind, and spirit. They served the twofold mission of "care for the body, cure for the soul," and would surround the bed and sing as one of their brothers was nearing their transition (Hollis, 2010, p.25).

The first time I played and sang for a patient during my clinical internship,[1] I was astounded at the intimacy of the experience. We were strangers to each other, and yet I was invited to bring my harp up close to Jim's hospital bed, right in the middle of the family room of his home. I observed his respiration and felt his pulse, noted the cast of his skin and the movement of his body. He was so sick. It was humbling to gaze into Jim's eyes, to visit briefly, to witness his frailty and his suffering. I invited him to simply rest and receive the music. I matched the rhythm of my playing with his breathing to create a subtle form of companioning. Vocals were added at times for another layer of human connection. I felt a deep sense of responsibility to lighten Jim's day, to provide solace perhaps, maybe ease his pain, and most of all honor his personhood with beauty in that moment. His sister was nearby in the kitchen, listening from a short distance.

End-of-life music aims to address what Cicely Saunders, a pioneer of modern hospice care, describes as "total pain—the suffering that encompasses all of a person's physical, psychological, social, spiritual and practical struggles" (Richmond, 2005).

My visits with patients, sometimes called vigils or music sessions, take place in private homes, hospice units, skilled nursing and assisted living facilities, and in various hospital units. Vigils are prescriptive in nature—a dynamic response to the patient's condition in the present moment—not a performance, but rather a therapeutic experience. My role is one of both an observer and participant, and while I enjoy making music, the work is intense.

On an icy day in Manhattan, I walked across Central Park to the hospital I was employed at that day. Experiencing the crunch of snow under my feet and the wind in my face was part of the centering practice that helped me prepare for the day ahead. I arrived on the hospice unit and asked the social

---

1   Names and details of people featuring in this chapter have been changed to provide anonymity.

worker if there were patients that would benefit from a music vigil. She said, "Yes. We have a patient who passed in the night. His parents are here, and they are refusing to leave the body. Nobody's been able to get them to go home."

I knocked on the door, entered, and caught my breath at the scene before me. The father, José, was standing at the head of the bed touching the handsome face of his deceased child. It was early in the day, and the morning light shone through the windows, casting a reflective glow on the walls and the white bedding. I sensed an other-worldly energy in the room. Today I can still see the 2 x 3-inch divine mercy prayer card that had been placed on the young person's chest. Liliana, his mother, sat slumped against the wall at the foot of the bed. She held a rosary in her hand. The parents looked at each other, then nodded their agreement to receive music. I brought the harp up close to the bed with the desire to bring honor, love, and solace to any aspects of life force that might linger. I began with melodies from the family's Catholic faith tradition, including lyrics sung in Latin. I chose songs that reside mostly in a minor key to acknowledge Liliana and José. José wanted to pay me, pulling cash out of his pants pocket. I quietly declined his generosity, bowed with palms together to the deceased patient, then bowed to the grieving parents before leaving the room. Within the hour, the nursing staff reported that the parents were headed home. The memory and mystery surrounding this music vigil is difficult to describe in words; it is one I will never forget.

I frequently exit a patient's hospital room to find a physician or other staff member lingering outside the door. A nurse told me that just hearing a few notes coming from the harp calmed him on stressful days, and he made a point of walking by the rooms where he knew a music vigil was taking place.

I provide bedside sessions for months, weeks, days, and even while the last breath is drawn. I am often invited to participate when someone is removed from life support. One day, I overheard the nurse practitioner quietly say to the team: "This always goes better when we have music." It is a time when loved ones need particular support, given that the outcome is anticipated but the specifics are unknown.

Last year, I received a voicemail from a hospice nurse regarding the husband of one of our former patients: "Bob is overcome with grief. I think a music session would really help him." It had been just two weeks since his wife's death. I called the bereaved husband to schedule a home visit, and he readily agreed. The couple had been married for many years. I offered my condolences upon arrival at their home and then invited Bob to make himself comfortable. He sat in his recliner, leaned back, and closed his eyes. The couch where his wife rested during my previous visits was empty. We spoke briefly about the depth of his pain since her passing. He said he had no idea it would be this hard.

I began with harp music in a minor key with long sustained base notes to meet the husband in his grief. Tears streamed down his face. When the music ended, Bob wiped his face, smiled, and said, "I do feel better. Thank you." His grief journey had just begun, but on this afternoon, he encountered a moment of relief. That was enough.

End-of-life music does not have the power to alter medical outcomes; however, it can change the energy in a room. The effects of a music session may include the relaxation of a patient's respiration and/or pulse. As their nervous system is calmed, they might also receive relief from pain, fear, agitation, or restlessness. Patients and family members sometimes fall into a deep sleep.

The music may allow family members to process the complexity and range of their feelings, from sadness, shock, and exhaustion to comfort and perhaps unity with the divine. Music sessions may provide loved ones with a memory of a peaceful exit, and this helps the survivor's bereavement process.

I provided a music vigil in the home of an elderly Mormon woman. It was a Sunday evening. She was unresponsive, and her vital signs reflected that she was actively dying. During the hour I was singing and playing my harp, the woman's five children, and over 20 grandchildren, and even great-grand-children—her entire posterity—came to her bedside and expressed heartfelt and teary goodbyes. It was an honor to witness so much love within the walls of that home.

The raw materials of music—melody, harmony, and rhythm—are friends in times of sorrow. Sound waves are translated by both the sensory-neural hearing (ears and brain) and conductive hearing (through porous skin and vibration of bones, body tissues, and organs). This means a person with hearing deficits can receive the benefits of music as an antidote to grief.

Not long ago, I played for a gentleman receiving hospice care in a hospital setting. His wife sat stoically at the foot of his bed while he slept. As soon as the music began, she started to weep, and she continued wiping her face throughout the session. At the conclusion of my visit, she said, "I don't usually let myself cry, but I couldn't help it when I heard the music. Thank you. I haven't been able to eat anything for days, but now I'm hungry." She pulled a sandwich out of her handbag and took a bite.

Creative Ways to Be with Music

My brother played his banjo at the bedside of our mother as Alzheimer's disease walked her toward the end of life. The banjo is clearly not a calming instrument of choice, but kudos to my brother who showed up with all of himself. He wanted to *do something* when faced with the inevitable death of his parent. The two of them were able to communicate without words. Mom smiled and laughed and waved other residents into her room during my brother's visits. Now I tease him since his other musical instrument is the saw, which is infinitely more annoying than the banjo.

> *The raw materials of music—melody, harmony, and rhythm—are friends in times of sorrow.*

Play an instrument. I learned to rely on playing the harp to help me through a hard time. If you are walking with grief, pick up an instrument, maybe one from your past, or consider learning a new one. Start slowly with just a few minutes a day, then increase the time as you can. Ask yourself how you feel at the end of a music-making session. Try to step away from self-judgment and just be with the sounds. Repetition enhances forward progress, so try to make time to practice each day. Taking private lessons is also a good idea, or check out the wealth of tutorials online. At some point, you may consider joining a band or orchestra for the added benefit of making music with others.

If you are providing music for a palliative or elderly patient, keep in mind that their skin is often thin, providing little protection from the outside world. Illness renders a person particularly vulnerable. Using a mute is a kindness to a fragile individual. Keep the volume lower than you would for a healthy person.

Create music with a synthesizer. Some grievers may find solace using a synthesizer to generate audio through various forms of analogue and digital technology. The creative possibilities are endless. A synthesizer is used in nearly every genre of music and is considered one of the most important instruments in the music industry. It is a perfect companion for a person who prefers to keep their own company in the wake of loss.

Offer or receive a virtual music session. One silver lining of the Covid-19 pandemic is that musicians have learned to provide remote music sessions for isolated patients via online video conferencing (Harps of Comfort, n.d.; Project: Music Heals Us, n.d.). The technology even allows the patient's loved ones to participate from another location. A cardiac patient at a hospital in the Midwest recently said to me at the end of a remote music vigil, "This is the most beautiful gift I've ever received." Then he kissed his fingers and touched them to the computer screen. The session was over. I set down the harp and closed my computer and my eyes, holding a mental screenshot of our last moment together and repeating his words in my mind. The gift goes both ways. Don't be afraid to experiment with the technology. The best sound settings are Original Sound on Zoom and Music Mode on Webex. Ask helpers on the patient's end to make sure you can see the recipient's face and upper torso via tablet or laptop in order to effectively connect with them.

Join a drum circle. The physicality of drumming meets a primal need to hit something—expressing anger, frustration, and more. A research study in the UK demonstrates that "group drumming provides a creative and mutual learning space in which mental health recovery can take place" (Perkins, 2016).

Attend a sound bath. Before the pandemic, I provided monthly sound baths at a New York City yoga studio alongside master gong player Michael Jay (Jay, n.d.). A sound bath is a meditative experience where those in attendance are "bathed" in sound waves to create a sense of harmony, relaxation, increased wellbeing, and expanded awareness. In addition to the harp and gong, Michael also brought his singing bowls, tuning forks, a shruti box, chimes, rattles, and more. We also sang. Attendees typically rest in the *savasana* (supine) position on a yoga mat with cushions and blankets. During sound baths, Michael and I often received audio waves from attendees that sounded a lot like snoring.

Use a singing bowl or tuning forks to create a sound massage for yourself. A study published in the *Journal of Evidence-Based Complementary and Alternative Medicine* looked at a group of 62 men and women and measured the levels of tension and overall mood before and after a Tibetan singing-bowl meditation. The results demonstrated that participants across the board experienced significantly less anxiety, tension, and fatigue and felt happier after the session (Goldsby, 2017). My daily meditation practice concludes with a few minutes of tuning-fork therapy because I am a sonic being and can easily get out of tune (Beaulieu, 2018).

Go to live concerts, including the opera and ballet. Live music is another version of a sound bath, whether it's a symphony or your favorite popular artist. I attended a Lady Gaga concert with my daughters where I could feel my body becoming entrained with the beat of the music. The bass track literally vibrated through me. It was a fabulous concert! It can feel good to be in community with others having the same experience. It can also feel overwhelming. I experienced both sensations that night.

The Healing Power of the Voice

The healing potential of the human voice is profound. Humming, chanting, toning, and singing all engage the vocal tract to process what is hurting in us. The vibrations restore a sense of balance to both body and mind because vocal production stimulates the vagus nerve, the largest nerve in the body. The vagus nerve connects the brain to major organs and sends messages to the brain that things are OK, or not. In *The Body Keeps the Score* (2014), Bessel Van der Kolk explains that the muscles of the face, throat, middle ear, and voice box or larynx communicate so effectively with the vagus nerve because of their close physical proximity to the brain stem.

Singing in a choir helped me through my first real experience with death. It was the summer of 1992 when my father suffered a heart attack and died very unexpectedly. I was bereft in the months that followed. Our family was living in Atlanta, Georgia at the time, and Pat Googe, the newly appointed choir director at the church we were attending, called and begged me to join. I initially turned her down, but she persisted until I reluctantly joined just in time to prepare for the Christmas program. My emotions felt raw and close to the surface that fall, and my tears flowed daily. Singing with the choir did not take away my sorrow, but for a few hours every week, I was deep in the music, concentrating intently, and distracted from my sadness. I was teary at times during the choir's big Christmas performance, mouthing the words when sound would not come out. I look back on that experience with deep gratitude for all the feelings and for the sense of community—breathing and sounding together—that helped me through that tender time.

Even singing along with a favorite recording connects us to the musical artist, to the evolution of that particular piece of music, and also to a larger community of fans, and we might feel less alone.

Chanting takes various forms. Generally speaking, it can be defined as the repetitive speaking or singing of words, phrases, or songs. Try attending a chanting session at your local yoga studio or meditation center where you might engage in a *kirtan*, a form of devotional singing originating in 15th-century India. The word derives from Sanskrit, meaning "praise eulogy." *Kirtan* relies on the repetition of a sung mantra in a call and response form. "With regular, sincere practice over time," says Grammy-winning artist Krishna Das, "you may notice that thoughts don't grab you so deeply. Emotions don't wipe you out so completely. It changes your psyche" (Kripalu, 2022). My experience with *kirtan* is of losing an awareness of time, which can be a balm for the bereaved.

I attended many chanting sessions on Sunday evenings with my Washington Heights meditation group, where we sang a Buddhist mantra 108 times to a simple melody. The practice becomes quite energetic, as you breathe and sound together. It was the perfect way to settle ourselves in preparation for a new week.

Ana Hernandez, author of *The Sacred Art of Chant* (2005), explains the benefits of chanting:

> Chant grounds and calms me, and if I'm tired, I can use it to raise my energy level; it opens me to things I find uncomfortable and painful in such a way that I'm able to work through the pain and discomfort.

Toning and humming. An individual who wants to find comfort and grounding can do so by elongating one long vowel tone at a time. This is toning. Start by choosing a pitch that is comfortably low to produce a "grounded, earthy, practical sense of well-being," suggests Joy Gardner-Gordon in *The Healing Voice* (Gardner-Gordon, 2005).

Peter Levine, in his book *In an Unspoken Voice* (2010), suggests using voo (rhymes with you) for therapeutic toning related to trauma. He describes how he introduces making the *voo* sound with clients:

> I often ask them to imagine a foghorn in a foggy bay sounding through the murk to alert ship captains that they are nearing land and to guide them safely home. This image works on different levels. First of all, the image of the fog represents the fog of numbness and dissociation. The foghorn represents the beacon that guides the lost boat (soul) back to safe harbor, to home in breath and belly... (p.126)

George W. Grant, author of *Zen in the Art of Vocal Toning* (2018), facilitates individual and group toning sessions online (Vocal Toning for Health, 2016). I have had the privilege of many in-person toning sessions with Grant, and I continue joining his online sessions because they are a self-regulating tonic during stressful times.

Humming is similar to toning, but the sound is made with closed lips, producing a wordless sound through the nose. Humming usually happens at a higher pitch than toning and can be very energizing.

Wisdom of Playlists

I recently dug through a box of old CDs to find a playlist that a dear friend had curated and downloaded onto a disk to support me during my season of loss. It is a delight today to listen to this playlist from yesteryear. I had lost touch with my friend when I moved to New York City but was inspired to reach out after finding the sonic treasure she had made. We both cried when I described unearthing the CD she had created years ago.

This experience reminds me of Rob Sheffield's memoir *Love Is a Mixtape* (2007) which beautifully illustrates the potency of a curated playlist. It is the story of the author and *Rolling Stone* magazine contributing editor Rob, and his girlfriend and later wife, Renee, making 22 mixtapes—sharing with each other their musical passion for rock and pop music. Renee tragically died of an embolism seven years after they met, and the tapes provided Rob with a priceless soundtrack for mourning her death.

Compiling a playlist for a friend or relative is a tangible act of love. A grieving person may not have the technological know-how or the energy, especially when their loss is recent. A custom playlist may assist a bereaved person in accessing their emotions, helping them rest when they are alone at night, filling the silence, and providing a much-needed companion. A playlist might distract a person from overwhelming grief or perhaps help them move their body when they feel up to it.

Online music services are powerful tools for curating a personalized soundscape as an acoustic safe space. If a grieving person randomly listens to the radio or to a streaming service on "shuffle" mode, a song may pop up that spontaneously triggers a wave of grief. Controlling the track selection is critical, particularly in the early stages after a loss. Some people will be comforted by listening to the favorite songs of their deceased loved one, while others may be upset. Talk about your playlist project with the intended recipient and ask what music they would like to have included. The "What's Your Grief?" website (Haley, 2022) provides a Spotify playlist of 74 songs that followers submitted as meaningful to them as grievers.

It is widely accepted that grief is not a linear process, nor is it a project with a fixed ending. Inviting music to accompany us on our grief journey is an opportunity to help make meaning along the way. Playlists related to Elisabeth Kübler-Ross's five stages of grief—anger, denial, bargaining, depression, acceptance—are also available online (Kübler-Ross, 1969).

Ambient music is a form of instrumental sound focusing on mood, tone, and texture, generally free of melody and rhythm. The spaciousness and variety of ambient music provides an opportunity to relax both mind and body. Brian Eno, British musician and composer, generally considered the father of ambient music, says in the liner notes from the release of *Ambient 1: Music for Airports* (Eno, 1978): "Ambient music must be able to accommodate many levels of listening attention without enforcing one in particular; it must be as ignorable as it is interesting." One of my favorite ambient albums is *Mixing Colours* by Brian and Roger Eno (Eno & Eno, 2020). I am drawn to it because it is a low-key musical conversation between brothers, a sound-painting that is a balm when I'm feeling anxious. More ambient music can be found online using search words such as spa, yoga, meditation, Zen, chill, relaxing, and new age music.

Isabelia Herrera, *New York Times* arts and music critic, wrote about the playlist of ambient music she compiled to comfort herself in the months after her mother's stroke. From her article "Ambient music isn't a backdrop. It's an invitation to suspend time" (2022), she writes:

> Time becomes supple, pliant, disobedient. Listening to it, I am forced to close my eyes, to feel the way that sound travels over the body, shapeshifting into nonlinear drift. I am detached from any deterministic version of the future. In this place between lightness and darkness, pleasure and pain exist in equal measure. I experience all the fragmentation of life, the reminders of trauma and uncertainty I have woken up to for the last four months. Here, I refuse to let grief become self-definition: I live unfettered from the speed of emergency.

Nature sounds. Recorded sounds of a rainstorm, wind blowing through trees, bird calls, or ocean waves are closely related to ambient music. Nature sounds may invite rest because they generally occur at a non-threatening low pitch and low volume, which may help to reduce the fight, flight, or freeze stress response.

Gregorian chant is an effective tool for the bereaved because it provides a horizontal stream of sound that can be an effective calming agent. Observation and self-reporting of elderly hospice patients indicates that listening to chant produces benefits to those with chronic illness by improving coping skills, quality of life, and overall sense of wellbeing (Twohey, 2013).

Gregorian chant came to be appreciated by a wide listening audience in the mid-1990s, with the release of *Chant* by the Benedictine Monks of Santo Domingo de Silos (1994). This form of chant developed mainly in Europe during the ninth and tenth centuries. It is typically defined by choirs of male or female voices singing a single melody line in unison, free of musical accompaniment. Unlike most Western music today, it is unmetered, meaning there is no time signature or strong downbeat. Melodies generally evolved to accommodate scriptural text, often from the Book of Psalms in the Old Testament. In addition to the *Chant* CD listed above, I recommend an album featuring female singers, *Voices: Chant from Avignon* (Benedictine Nuns of Notre-Dame de L'Assonciation, 2010), be added to your chant playlist.

Sad music is loosely defined by music in minor keys, while songs in a major key generally convey a happier mood. Professor David Huron, a researcher in the field of music cognition, explores the science of sad sounds. He says that listening to sad music causes the body to release prolactin, which "has a consoling psychological effect—it's like mother nature is sort of wrapping her arms around you and consoling you and saying 'there-there everything is okay' and you have this warm fuzzy feeling" (Huron, 2010). Samuel Barber's *Adagio for Strings* in B-flat minor is the first selection I would choose for a playlist of sad music.

Listening to sad music is an example of a homeopathic remedy or iso music therapy principle (Heiderscheidt, 2015) wherein the music matches the patient's or the mourner's mood. The key, lyrics, pitch, and sense of movement mirror what we are feeling. When the music conveys emotions similar to ours, we may feel as though we're not grieving alone. Sad music reminds us that suffering and sorrow are part of the universal human experience.

A sad music playlist validates our feelings, and it may open the door to a release of deep emotion. Physician and writer Judith Orloff discusses the beneficial aspects of crying on her website (Orloff, 2017). She says, "Crying makes us feel better, even when a problem persists. In addition to physical detoxification, emotional tears heal the heart. You don't want to hold tears back."

Popular music. Favorite music, usually popular songs from a patient's youth, can be a source of comfort to both declining patients and survivors. A playlist of someone's favorite songs is a sonic personal history and is useful in commemorating the life of the person who has died. Several years ago, at the luncheon following a high school friend's memorial service, the soundtrack of songs by James Taylor and Carole King was the most meaningful aspect of the entire day for me. This is when the memories of my deceased friend bubbled up, and I was transported to a moment when we sat next to each other listening to these same tunes as teenagers.

Music to invite movement. Physical movement has long been a known antidote to mental anguish. Listening to up-tempo music might inspire a grieving person to move their body, which might help them process stored emotions. Movement increases heart and respiration rates, bringing oxygen to the brain and body.

Lyn Prashant—somatic thanatologist and death, dying, and bereavement educator and counselor—writes in the foreword of Antonio Sausys' *Yoga for Grief Relief* (Prashant, 2012, p.xii):

> As an athlete, physical education teacher, and coach I saw how the physical body not only needs its own expression but actually demands physical release. This resets the balance of the many interconnected complex biological systems involved in grief. My thinking was clearer after a run, or a dance, or a swim. I saw that when I engaged my body, I felt energized rather than drained. I was feeling a life force inside of me resurging.

Paul Denniston's Grief Yoga workshops are magical. I've experienced them in real life and also streamed via the internet. Paul's compassionate approach, coupled with a beautifully curated soundtrack, helps participants transform pain and struggle into a sense of peace and purpose. The free resources on Paul's website are a gift to anyone who might not know how or where to begin moving (Denniston, 2021).

Whether one creates a playlist to encourage exercise or engages with an inspired teacher, coach, or program, moving the body helps us bear the unbearable. The first steps out of a state of immobility related to the trauma of loss may be the biggest steps we ever take. Music helps us take them.

Note: Recorded music should not be left looping in the room of a sick patient. They may not have the capacity to either turn it off themselves or tell you when they've had enough. An hour of recorded music at one time is plenty. Silence is a friend.

Music as Final Honoring Ritual

I provided background music for a family that was saying goodbye to an infant daughter, a victim of sudden infant death syndrome. There was not a dry eye in the room, including mine. I played the harp while witnessing the parents hold and kiss the body of their child for the last time. I believe that the grieving family will have memories of that day, including a soundtrack of curated lullabies that supported them during that extraordinarily painful moment.

Music as a vehicle for grief rituals takes many forms. The children of the American abstract artist Mark Rothko slipped two of his favorite cassette tapes into the casket before the lid was closed. Classical recordings of works by Schubert and Mozart were the audio heartbeat of his studio, and sending their dad off with the tapes he loved was a meaningful gesture to his children (Comenas, 2016).

Music softens the edges at wakes, funerals, memorial and graveside services, and other end-of-life rituals. It adds to the symbolic dimension of the final disposition of the body and plays an important role in helping attendees along their mourning path. This is the last interaction with a loved one in physical form.

Playing *Greensleeves* at my father's funeral was something I needed to do in order to feel complete. He is the one who drove me to harp lessons each Saturday morning, and he was often a presence in my practice room just reading or writing at the desk across the room. Dad had no formal music training, which made him the perfect audience. I could count on his asking me to play *Greensleeves* for all visitors to our home. And so I played it for him one last time.

Musical choices evoke a sense of the spiritual, regardless of whether a funeral takes place within a church or is guided by a faith tradition or none at all. Today there is much more flexibility for next of kin to create a ritual to express the character of their deceased loved one and perhaps engage music to conjure shared memories.

People attending a wake or other memorializing event are emotionally open, with the masks they wear in everyday life set aside. A bereaved person often doesn't have the energy to be anything but their unvarnished self. Their heart seems open to receiving the music in a way that is much different from attendees at a wedding or party.

How does a family go about choosing music for their loved one's final honoring ritual? The internet provides endless lists of favorite funeral music depending on personal preferences related to faith tradition, genre, and the age of the deceased. If clergy are involved, they will have suggestions and perhaps provide a traditional format such as a funeral mass or traditional hymns to support grieving friends and families.

Final Thoughts

Music illuminates what is alive in us. It transcends worlds, lifting us up when we are down and opening us up to our core feelings. Vocal or instrumental sound—live or recorded—is a sublime gift to both the living and the dying at every stage of the process. It is a privilege to be able to help individuals as they are winding down, and also to honor the bereavement process with music when they are gone.

Each one of us can engage sound in some form as a vehicle for helping ourselves and others to be with our grief. This might involve planning a meaningful memorial service, listening to curated playlists, humming, or singing in a choir. Whatever approach we take, the true nature of loss and suffering is made more bearable when we are held by music.

References

Beaulieu, J. (2018). *Sound Healing and Values Visualization: Creating a Life of Value*. High Falls, NY: BioSonic Enterprises.

Benedictine Monks of Santo Domingo de Silos (1994). *Chant*. Madrid: Angel Records.

Benedictine Nuns of Notre-Dame de L'Assonciation (2010). *Voices: Chant from Avignon*. Avignon: Decca Records.

Comenas, G. (2016). Abstract Expressionism 1970–1974. Warholstars.org. https://warholstars. org/abstract-expressionism/timeline/mark_rothko.html

Denniston, P. (2021). Grief Yoga: free resources. https://griefyoga.com

Eno, B. (1978). *Ambient 1: Music for Airports*. London: Polydor Records.

Eno, B. & Eno, R. (2020). *Mixing Colours*. Deutsche Grammaphon.

Gardner-Gordon, J. (2005). *The Healing Voice: Traditional and Contemporary Toning, Chanting and Singing*. Woodstock, VT: Skylight Paths Publishing.

Goldsby, T.G. (2017). Effects of singing bowl sound meditation on mood, tension and well-being: An observational study. *Journal of Evidence-Based Complementary and Alternative Medicine, 22*(3), 401–406. https://doi.org/10.1177%2F2156587216668109

Grant, G. (2018). *Zen in the Art of Vocal Toning—For Energy and Empowerment*. Self-published.

Haley, E. (2022). What's Your Grief Lyric? What's Your Grief. https://whatsyourgrief.com/what-is-your-grief-lyric

Harps of Comfort (n.d.). About us: Harps of Comfort offers remote music to patients and their loved ones. www.harpsofcomfort.com

Heiderscheidt, A. (2015). Use of the iso principle as a central method in mood management: A music psychotherapy clinical case study. *Music Therapy Perspectives, 33*(1), 45–52. http://dx.doi.org/10.1093/mtp/miu042

Hernandez, A. (2005). *The Sacred Art of Chant: Preparing to Practice*. Woodstock, VT: Skylight Paths Publishing.

Herrera, I. (2022). Ambient music isn't a backdrop. It's an invitation to suspend time. *The New York Times*, April 14. www.nytimes.com/2022/04/14/arts/music/ambient-music.html

Hollis, J.L. (2010). *Music at the End of Life: Easing the Pain and Preparing the Passage*. Santa Barbara, CA: Praeger.

Huron, D. (2010). The science of sad sounds. YouTube. www.youtube.com/watch?v=_pwqBAS9x3U&ab_channel=TheNationalNews

Jay, M. (n.d.). Michael Jay Sound. www.michaeljaysound.com/about

Jenny, H. (2001). *Cymatics: A Study of Wave Phenomena and Vibration*. Newmarket, NH: Macromedia Press.

Kripalu. (2022). The beginners' guide to kirtan and mantra. https://kripalu.org/resources/beginners-guide-kirtan-and-mantra

Kübler-Ross, E. (1969). *On Death and Dying: What the Dying Have to Teach Doctors, Nurses, Clergy and Their Own Families*. New York, NY: Scribner.

Levine, P. (2010). *In an Unspoken Voice: How the Body Releases Trauma and Restores Goodness*. Berkeley, CA: North Atlantic Books.

Orloff, J. (2017). The healing power of tears. https://drjudithorloff.com/the-healing-power-of-tears

Perkins, R.A. (2016). Making music for mental health: How group drumming mediates healing. *Psychology of Well Being, 6*, 11. https://doi.org/10.1186/s13612-016-0048-0

Prashant, L. (2012). Foreword. In A. Sausys, *Yoga for Grief Relief: Simple Practices for Transforming Your Grieving Mind and Body*. Oakland, CA: New Harbinger.

Project: Music Heals Us (n.d.). Mission. www.pmhu.org

Richmond, C.S. (2005). Obituaries: Dame Cicely Saunders. *British Medical Journal, 331*, 238. https://doi.org/10.1136/bmj.331.7510.238

Schroeder-Sheker, T. (2001). *Transitus: A Blessed Death in the Modern World*. Baltimore, MD: St. Dunstan's Press.

Sheffield, R. (2007). *Love Is a Mixtape: Life and Loss One Song at a Time*. New York, NY: Three Rivers Publishing.

Twohey, A. (2013). The Effects of Plainchant on Subjective Measures of Emotions and Heart Rate Variance. *Honors Theses, 1963–2015*, 1. https://digitalcommons.csbsju.edu/honors_theses/1

Van der Kolk, B. (2014). *The Body Keeps the Score: Mind, Brain and Body in the Transformation of Trauma*. New York, NY: Penguin.

Vocal Toning for Health (2016). About George Grant. https://vocaltoning.net/about-george-grant

All This

A metallic gray mist slid,
circling the silvered peaks,
rising slow,
piercing the electric halo.

On the dark side of night,
earth spinning
at the speed of light
in a vortex of shadow.

At the end of the
narrowing corridor of day,
the dark has a distinct shape,
slanted and unbalanced.

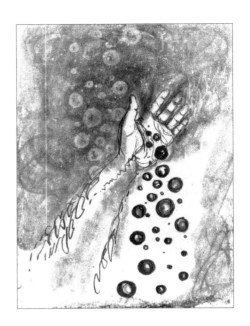

It cast its spell,
eclipsed the moon,
a silent tide slipping and sliding
in purple and blues.

All this...on the day you died
and children's toys
lying scattered about the floor.

All this...
on the day you died
All this...
nothing more.

~ Steven "Mud" Roues

CHAPTER 5

Pleasure and the Senses in the Grief Journey

Oceana Sawyer

Grief is messy. There is nothing linear or rational about it. There is not even a beginning, a middle, and an end. Also, just forget about any stages.

What I know about grief came first when I discovered that my mother, whom I loved dearly and was a cultural anchor in my life, was going to die within a few months. She had started to make seemingly casual comments asking if I knew where all her accounts were in case she didn't wake up in the morning, or if I thought my brother was going to make it through life without her support. Initially, I brushed aside those comments with breezy replies asserting the positive. As they began to occur more frequently and with a slowly growing intensity, it dawned on me she might be telling me that she was going to die soon. When I factored in her reduced interest in leaving the house and reduced appetite, I made a plan to go along with her the next time she mentioned her impending death. From the time I came to that conclusion until the time she gave me another opportunity was only a few days. "So, let's suppose you are dying, how would you like it to go?" was my reply to one of her casual comments. Far from denying it, she simply looked at me directly in the eyes and grunted an approval. No further words were uttered on the topic that day, but from that moment we both shared a reality, and that changed everything.

I immediately felt profound grief, even though she hadn't yet died. Called anticipatory grief, it is quite common, particularly among caregivers. This is the grief that occurs when you know a death is imminent. It could be called pre-grieving; however, that is not quite accurate. Because along with anticipating a coming loss, there can be secondary losses that occur along the way to a big loss. These losses include diminished physical and mental capacity, a change in status related to employment, family role, friendships, or community standing; and losses related to finances. Any of these and more can activate anticipatory grief.

This type of grief can be just as challenging as any other type of grief. It comes with a variety of modes of presentation similar to general grief, including the inability to concentrate, lethargy, irritation, anxiety, random bouts of crying, and a range of others. Because anticipatory grief is not commonly recognized, you may get responses from people that indicate you are over-reacting because no one has died yet. This can be devastating at worst, while at best it can feel like gaslighting.

I certainly had the experience of confusion and lethargy. I also withdrew from my own life as my mother's needs grew and I moved further into the realm of death as I companioned her on the journey to the end of her life.

Throughout the process, I had been training as a death doula so that I could help others negotiate those waters.

I had also been a sensualist for many years, which provided me a unique perspective on bodily sensation and physical pleasure,[1] which I believe is a healing force. It was through these lenses, and within a supportive community, that I came to experience genuine curiosity about the grief process. It occurred to me that my mother's dying, and her subsequent death, could be a unique opportunity for maturation if I was willing to surrender to the big, complicated process that is available as one tends to the dying process and the resulting grief.

Knowing myself as I do, I knew that the degree of surrender I sought would be most possible via my own physicality; or, rather, via my own capacity to feel and process with my senses: in other words, my sensuality.

Metabolizing the Energy of Emotions

For me, this type of physical expression is not only an effective way to metabolize the energy of my emotions; the release of that energy is also something I often experience as enjoyable. A good example of this is a long run after a stressful day at work, or putting on your favorite music and dancing ferociously after sitting through an intense Zoom call. Moving heavy, stagnant energy through one's body can be a relief at the most visceral level.

---

[1] I define physical pleasure as the expression of emotion through the body in a way that feels good.

This experience of pleasure at the most challenging transitions in life is something I fell into after experiencing the intense loss of my mother.

It was natural for me to find information about and express my own grief through my body. The initial foray into my body looking for grief involved literally carving out a few moments to just be still long enough to notice and feel my body before I could even get to the actual feelings. My preferred modality was to sit outside in the sun with my eyes closed for a few minutes with my attention on my breath and a bit of curiosity about what sensations were occurring in my body. For instance, I would ask myself what the tightness in my chest was about or what this hollow sensation was, in the bottom of my stomach. I let this inquiry unfold gently. In the initial stages, I often had to remind myself to just allow something authentic to emerge and resist the urge to make up a familiar or convenient story about what the sensations meant.

We humans can be quite proficient at meaning making. However, the body is a much more feral realm than the mind. It requires a spaciousness of time and a certain amount of discipline to drop conditioned patterns of over-thinking and just allow the body to inform and guide the inquiry into grief.

All this is made more difficult as much of the mourning period, the first phase of active grieving, is about the logistics of after-death management. Busyness can also become an effective strategy for avoiding the intense feelings of loss. Socially, it is very easy to continue in this mode of appearing occupied so you can tell everyone what they desperately want to hear, which is that you are fine.

Creating Space for Grief

Creating enough physical and mental space to just *be* can feel daunting, especially if you imagine it as something that requires a special trip somewhere and possibly an outlay of money. Spending money is definitely an option, but it is also completely unnecessary, particularly if it provides yet another excuse not to tend to yourself. As indicated earlier, it doesn't require much more than pausing for five minutes in your car before you go in the house or going out into your yard or the balcony for a few minutes with no agenda except to be. You don't even have to be absolutely still. Paying attention to your breath, swaying, stretching, closing your eyes are small activities that don't provide as much distraction as they offer an entry into your body and how it feels.

Another route is to do your normal physical activity with a bit more attention. If you take walks in the morning or swim laps in the afternoon, adding in more attention to how you are breathing or moving, or noticing what feels heavy or constricted, are also opportunities to use your tactile sense to touch into where grief might be living in your body. Once you have access, you can use more of your senses to excavate further. If you begin with putting a hand on your belly and notice a ball of heat there, you could explore what tastes might be alive in your mouth in that moment. That might lead you to a memory that unlocks a release of the heat in your belly.

Swimming, sex, walks in nature, culinary adventures, acupuncture, body-work, and music were all sources of healing for me. They each provided a body-based sensory avenue that allowed me to touch into different aspects of my grief well enough that metabolization was possible. What I mean by metabolization in this context is when a specific experience of grief becomes something else, most likely an emotional experience that feels less heavy and more easily digestible, nourishment for the body and psyche, an insight. I also worked with an online grief therapist for the periods when I wanted to do some cognitive integration. It can be very useful to have a multi-pronged approach.

The confluence of all these factors—my commitment to consciously opening to the entirety of my experience, my sensual approach to the process, the support from my community and husband, and a bit of therapy—enabled me to experience my grief as a spacious, natural, and raw entity that wanted, in the most genuine and purest sense, to be felt.

For me, grief is an entity that has its own life and flow. Its boundaries are more permeable than those of a human being or animal. It wants to be known. The porosity of grief makes it far more accessible than perhaps is imagined. In fact, the vehicle of the senses allows for more of a multidimensional experience with grief, making it remarkably knowable in a sense. As close as our very breath, there is an intimacy to grief that is similar to death except that it is survivable.

The Importance of Grieving

In my work with people on a grief journey, I strive to create a container that activates at least two of the senses, most often sound in the form of live crystal bowls or specially chosen music, and the tactile sense in the form of placing one hand on the heart and the other on the belly while rocking or swaying gently. The visual senses are also often engaged in the form of resting the eyes on something pleasing in one's immediate environment. These are all ways that I create a space where grievers can disconnect from their judging mind that wants to assess if they are doing it right, and instead enter into their body with more ease.

It is often in this relatively unfamiliar place (because we spend so much time in our heads) that I experience people contacting their grief for the first time in some cases, and freshly in other cases. In both instances, the process often results in a revelatory experience with grief, one that has the unique potential to integrate and inform the griever with new emotional insights and likely a sense of wellbeing as well.

The Dagara people of West Africa are quite familiar with grief in this way. For them, the entire life cycle is a series of rituals that involve the community in a full-bodied approach to the significant transitions in life. It should be further noted that they don't really have the Western European concept of the individual. What is occurring for one individual is occurring to some degree for every person and being in the village or community. In that context, grief occurs as another aspect of the life cycle that must be tended to by the entire community. Sobonfu Somé, African ritualist, teacher, and author, sums it up:

> For my people, the Dagara tribe of Burkina Faso in West Africa, we see that in life it is necessary to grieve those things that no longer serve us and let them go. When I grieve I am surrounded by family reassuring me that the grieving is worthwhile and I can grieve as much as I want. We experience conflicts, loved ones die or suffer, dreams never manifest, illnesses occur, relationships break up, and there are unexpected natural disasters. It is so important to have ways to release those pains to keep clearing ourselves. Hanging on to old pain just makes it grow until it smothers our creativity, our joy, and our ability to connect with others. It may even kill us. Often my community uses grief rituals to heal wounds and open us to spirit's call. (Somé, n.d.)

In another undated interview, Somé makes a point of mentioning how important it is to metabolize grief in somatic ways that include crying and walking in nature to allow the body an opportunity to recover from the loss so that a sense of safety and sanity is restored. The grief rituals in the Dagara communities involve several days of communal wailing, dancing, drumming, singing, feasting, and ceremony. This type of ritual is known to be an important aspect of individual and communal development.

The felt sense of grief can be so rich when encountered in this way. As a result of this kind of experience, it's possible to perceive some bit of sweetness, almost a benevolence, previously unknown. Amid even the pulpiest moments, it can envelop the griever like a blanket, sometimes warm and often heavy. This certainly was my experience, and it surely colored the interactions I had with other people. The warmth allowed for openness while the heaviness sparked alternately irritation and compassion. These unfamiliar states would cause confusion and then judgment. Still, the magnitude of the loss often led me back to compassion for others and a tenderness for my body which seemed to be holding so much.

The first few weeks after my mother's death were a whirlwind of activity, yet I experienced them in slow motion, a kind of time out of time, which allowed me to slow down enough to truly be with loved ones and my own experience. The uniqueness of the portal that grief can open up cannot be under-estimated.

This term "grief portal" came to me on a walk with a fellow griever. I was describing to her how an image had come to me in the middle of a cryfest. Out of a gray mist came a charcoal-gray smoke ring that slowly grew until it revealed an opening. I had unknowingly passed through the portal at some point earlier, most likely around the time of my mother's dying. The ring appeared only to reveal to me that I was in a particular place and that there was an exit which I could choose whenever I was ready. Knowing that I had a choice made all the difference. Then I could just be in the space and enjoy the unfolding experience that gets opened up when someone leaves this world and passes to the next.

This is also a space that lends itself to a gentle kind of exploration around what actually feels good and nourishes you on multiple levels as you settle into grief and allow it to have its way with you.

Movement—in this case, walking—was so useful to me in terms of grounding a big new experience in my body, providing another avenue to process or metabolize the experience.

Feeling the hard earth below your feet and a breeze on your face can be settling in a way that allows for access to more ways of knowing.

In my book *Life, Death, Grief, and the Possibility of Pleasure*, Naila Francis describes how she accesses various aspects of her grief via walking in the natural world:

To step out into nature is to move my body with a rhythm that says, you, too, are of earth. It is to carry water. Know how to bend and flow. Sometimes I hum. Sometimes a song floats from the trees, the sky, bubbles up on my lips. I welcome any expression, make myself available to praise, to marvel… not instead of sorrow, but as companions. A way to drink in the world, stay open to more than the bleeding, the sting. To notice how my body makes room, is more spacious, always more spacious, than my grief would have me believe. (Sawyer, 2022)

Pandemic, Racial, and Gender-based Grief

After the death of my mother, the coronavirus exploded onto the scene, quickly followed by the ignition of a racial awakening/reckoning. Both of these physically impactful and horrific circumstances further expanded and deepened the experience of grief in my world. With so many of my normal distractions suddenly unavailable to me, I leaned into what seemed familiar and accessible, which turned out to be meditation and gentle forms of yoga. They soothed me well enough. I also utilized books, podcasts, and workshops that had a somatic focus. In those early days of the twin pandemics, it was the body that seemed particularly reactive while faithfully witnessing in captivity the relentless news cycles displaying so much violence to other bodies—specifically and primarily, bodies that were racialized Black or Brown (Latinx, Asian, Indigenous).

The relentless impact of systemic racism in the medical and law enforcement institutions was revealed in seeming Technicolor, which created a condition among those directly affected that could only be described as compounded or cumulative grief. This occurs when a person experiences multiple losses that may occur in close chronology or over the span of a lifetime. The key factor is that none of the losses has been adequately processed.

The truth is that nearly everyone experienced some form of cumulative grief in 2020. However, the experience was particularly acute for people in racialized and gender-expansive[2] bodies. The fact that these experiences of

---

2   Gender-expansive is "an umbrella term sometimes used to describe people who expand notions of gender expression and identity beyond perceived or expected societal norms. Some gender-expansive individuals identify as a mix of genders, some identify more binarily as a man or a woman, and some identify as no gender." National Institutes of Health. www.edi.nih.gov/people/sep/lgbti/safezone/terminology

loss and trauma centered on particular types of bodies suggests that somatic methodologies for processing cumulative grief might be most effective.

Indeed, that was my experience. One approach that I found particularly effective for myself and with other bodies of culture (aka people of the global majority or popularly as people of color) was the somatic abolitionist work of Resmaa Menakem, who wrote *My Grandmother's Hands* (2017). In it, he offers a set of body-based practices for metabolizing historic, intergenerational, persistent institutional, and personal (HIPP) trauma. These practices also worked well for processing the grief so many people in BOC[3] continue to experience.

Fatal violence against transgender and gender non-conforming people disproportionately affects people of color. Since 2013, at least 85 percent of victims of violence against transgender and gender non-conforming people were people of color. In 2020, 22 victims were Black and seven were Latinx, of which 25 were Black or Latinx women (Brown, 2021).

Much more can be said on this topic, but it's fair to say that embodied grieving methodologies have the double benefit of allowing the most socially vulnerable people not only to process cumulative grief, but also to metabolize intergenerational racialized trauma in the form of somatic practices.

In this regard, Arielle Schwartz captures how important the body is to the grief journey in this blog post that she wrote in February 2016 entitled "Healing grief and loss":

> Not all grieving is painful. As you adjust to loss you might begin to make new choices, forge new relationships, or discover new aspects of yourself. You may discover unexpected strengths, renew hope, and even find a desire to help others. (Schwartz, 2016)

The practices that she offers are similar to those that Menakem indicates in *My Grandmother's Hands*. Here is a practice that I use with my own clients.

After you find a comfortable position and begin to attune to the emotional terrain within your body, you might experiment with this practice which I use with groups to become comfortable with experiencing big emotions in the body:

---

3   BOC—Bodies of Culture—is a term coined by Resmaa Menakem in his book *My Grandmother's Hands*.

Notice your breath. Does it seem tight and shallow or full and easy? Where does it feel constricted? What part of your body is actually occupying?

Do not change anything at first. You need only bring your relaxed curiosity. There is nothing to fix because nothing is wrong. You're just exploring for a few minutes.

Start to notice how your attention is changing your breathing, if at all.

Shift your attention to the area of your body that feels the most constricted, and gently move your breath to that area. Let your breath be as a beloved friend asking, "How are you doing? What's going on here?"

Pause and allow a response to float up into your consciousness. Keep breathing normally.

Try placing one of your hands or any body part on the area that feels constricted. You may be receiving information about the grief in that area, and touch can be soothing at that point. Experiment with the pressure or even a movement that feels especially good.

You can also adjust your breathing to bring additional calming to the restricting area. Deeper breaths with longer exhales are especially effective. Be curious and explore what feels the best for you moment to moment.

Finish up the practice with a gentle rocking motion from your torso in any direction.

You can use your breath to generate a humming sound, which is particularly effective for metabolizing grief.

Take as long as you need to explore deeply and allow whatever feelings arise to have their due. These experiences often have an arc: they build and subside naturally.

Given the well-known connection between grief and the lungs, it's little wonder that this form of breathing, specifically pranayama, became a potent resource for locating and metabolizing grief within my body and psyche. Many cultures have information related to where grief is stored in the body. The people of China and India locate grief in the lungs.

Pranayama is a Sanskrit term that means breath or vital life force energy (prana) that is controlled in order to create an expansion (yama or ayama). Pranayama is simply a technique to control the breath for the purpose of expanding one's consciousness. In Traditional Chinese Medicine, the function of the lungs is to take in new energy and release old energy. Not being able to release energy fully from the lungs is associated with the emotions of grief. Of course, these are very simple definitions of two very complex energetic systems, neither of which I can claim to have studied in any depth.

However, these two systems do offer a plausible context for what occurred for me when I sat down to a guided practice with a leading yoga teacher. The breath exercises she led me in quickly became a tidal wave of pent-up sorrow released from my body in the form of gasps and tears.

One of the yoga teachers that I followed in the initial phase of my grief journey was Sara Clark, who is a popular yoga teacher based in New York City. In a virtual breathwork class I took from her in the early days of the coronavirus pandemic, which happened to coincide with my mother's passing, Clark talked about her own experience of grief and how her yoga practice supported her. She explained:

> And so now, I have an opportunity to mindfully tend to my grief, to not pour myself back into work so quickly like I did after each visit. To instead water myself like I do my plants.
>
> Because...the anticipation of grief is still here. But it's no longer about the loss, it's about how my heart will handle it...how my family will handle it. And this is where the practice begins again. So I am unplugging this week to be in my practice. To float in the spaciousness that loss brings. The tenderness. The breath. The little moments that mean everything. I need to be supple for the energetic recalibration that is underway.

Although the onslaught of emotion brought on by the twin tidal waves of Covid-19 and the violence against Black bodies was at times as overwhelming for me as it was for so many, I felt largely tethered. Even in the aftermath of my mother's death, I mostly felt grounded. Big emotions—outrage and helplessness and terror—swept through me, yes. But I was present to them. I was with them with all of my body, all of my energy. And so, much of the time, instead of feeling drowned by my tears and internal (and external) screams, I was able to ride them. Surf them.

The editors of the *Yoga Journal* offer these tips for practice from an October 2014 article entitled "The yoga sequence for a healing heart," which mirrors my own practice:

> Find the inner strength to process grief and loss this season with this yoga sequence, which calls on chest-opening lunges, backbends, and twists;

nurturing restorative poses; and a focus on moving slowly with your breath. The more active postures keep energy moving in the heart, while the restorative poses give your central nervous system the opportunity to rest, which can relieve some of the deep fatigue that often accompanies grief. Practice every morning in a quiet, private space.

Throughout the sequence, put your physical sensations into words: "tense," "tired," "heavy." Then name your emotions, too: "heartbroken," "angry," "scared." This helps you to be present so you can begin to heal, instead of shutting down or running away from your grief and prolonging your heartbreak. Remember to exhale fully to release physical and emotional tension. (YJ Editors, 2014)

This sensation of being with difficult emotions, I came to realize, truly is the body at its holiest.

At its realest. At its truest. And, thus, at its most pleasured. For pleasure as I'm defining it doesn't exclude pain. Rather, true pleasure is the conscious, *felt* integration of every emotion through the body—and those emotions very much include the large, difficult, and most painful ones—the ones we most want to push away.

And here's the beauty of that integration: the more pain you are able to truly, consciously feel and integrate through the body, the more pleasure, the more awe, the more glory you are able to truly, consciously feel and integrate through the body as well.

Taking Care of the Dying

My recent experiences with grief have led me to a rather stunning conclusion: that body-centered death care encompassing pleasure can increase a dying person's capacity for personal expansion. It's an idea that is redefining my work as a death doula.

The point of comfort-centric death care is to ensure the dying person is in as little pain as possible. A noble and vitally important and compassionate goal, yes, but with pleasure-centric death care, we can focus further than the objective of pain reduction. We can aim for the dying person—and their caregivers—to feel as good as possible throughout the death process.

A helpful starting point is understanding pleasure as a potential source of energy. For instance, it is not uncommon for many people to respond to a lengthy, draining meeting by "taking a break." They may choose to refresh their beverage or go to the bathroom, and along the way they catch a glimpse of blue sky through a window, or they walk outside for a couple of minutes to "clear their head" by feeling the breeze on their skin. These are all mini-energy boosters by way of accessing pleasure in the form of a sensual stimulus that the person has judged feels good to them. Pleasure is a source of energy that gives them the fuel to go on with the meeting.

Moreover, it is likely that this act of gathering renewed energy also brings with it a new idea or thought for how to proceed in the meeting in which they are involved. Head clearing is another way of saying you are releasing old thoughts to make space for new ones. Similarly, pleasure is beneficial in the arduous task of winding down a life. By including elements in the dying process that go beyond comfort, there is the possibility for divine inspiration and/or guidance. An example would be closing the door to a dying person's hospital room, turning off the lights (with agreement from the staff), and playing the dying person's favorite music, particularly something of a spiritual or religious nature if that suits them. Given that many believe that hearing is the last sense to go, this act has every possibility of moving the dying person in the direction of beliefs that can support them in the process. It also has the ancillary benefit of giving the loved ones present something pleasant on which to put their attention, allowing them more access to the generative emotions of love and care which they can then impart to the person who is passing.

This can be especially useful in situations in which the dying person and their family and/or friends have become depleted from navigating institutional medical oppression. Just getting basic medical and comfort care can be a challenge, but once that is achieved, it makes sense to lean into whatever feels good as a way to restore the human right to die as well as possible. For people of African descent, these are time-honored ways that allowed us to survive the horrors of enslavement.

Thus, more felt pleasure creates more energy, more buoyancy, so that a dying person can more nimbly navigate the many vicissitudes of that process. When we have more pleasure-based energy in our bodies, we are empowered—we literally have more power—to handle difficulties with greater grace.

Alice Walker says it beautifully in *Hard Times Require Furious Dancing*:

Though we have all encountered our share of grief and troubles, we can still hold the line of beauty, form, and beat—no small accomplishment in a world as challenging as this one. Hard times require furious dancing. Each of us is the proof. (Walker, 2013, p.16)

In my practice, my primary goal is always to ensure that the wishes of the person dying are met, first and foremost. Then I do what I can to alleviate suffering. Embedded in all of that is an eye toward the ultimate goal of allowing for the kind of end-of-life experience that has the possibility of transformation for everyone involved. That is where pleasure becomes useful.

The Holiness of Grief and Pleasure

Pleasure can also be effective in the grieving process in the same way. Grief is often defined as the pain or sorrow associated with loss. However, anyone who has really embraced their grieving will say it is also so much more than that. Currently, many practitioners describe grief as a range of emotions, behaviors, and physiological experiences that ebb and flow, undulate, and meander. In other words, grief is a journey—a journey of huge emotions. And it can become a grand adventure if we are willing to honor those emotions by feeling them fully through our bodies. When we dare to feel fully, we feel *good*. Righteously so. For instance, a big old howling, screaming sobfest can feel exquisite at any point in the act, if it's embraced and cherished as the soul-nourishing act that it is.

Grieving becomes an elevated, sacred rite when we are willing to do this—willing to fully feel all of what wants to come through. We become aware of our majestic capacity for emotion, our infinite capacity to love. We are rendered more deeply human, more fully ourselves, more at home within Ourselves.

Grieving becomes an elevated, sacred rite when we are willing to do this—willing to fully feel all of what wants to come through. We become aware of our majestic capacity for emotion, our infinite capacity to love. We are rendered more deeply human, more fully ourselves, more at home *within* ourselves. We have accessed the sheer space and permission to have all that is available to be felt and thus transform an experience of heavy stuckness into something life-affirming and possibly even transcendent.

The concepts of the body, feeling, pleasure, and death—and large, unwieldy, and inconvenient emotions—do not go together in our society. We isolate them from each other. I believe we do so to our detriment. I also believe, though, that if we take a more holistic, open, and less fearful approach to death, and if we are bold enough to reimagine what the death experience, and grief and outrage and even fear, can look like, then we have the capacity to truly expand our human potential for spiritual elevation. And we can do so right here, right now, in our very own humble—and very holy—bodies.

References

Brown, J.C. (2021). An epidemic of violence: Fatal violence against transgender and gender non-conforming people in the United States in 2020. Human Rights Campaign Foundation: https://reports.hrc.org/an-epidemic-of-violence-fatal-violence-against-transgender-and-gender-non-confirming-people-in-the-united-states-in-2021

Menakem, R. (2017). *My Grandmother's Hands*. Las Vegas, NV: Central Recovery Press.

Sawyer, O. (2022). *Life, Death, Grief, and the Possibility of Pleasure*. Good to Be Better.

Schwartz, A. (2016). Healing grief and loss. Center for Resilience Informed Therapy, February 22. https://drarielleschwartz.com/healing-grief-and-loss-dr-arielle-schwartz/#.Yqooty-cZUc

Somé, S. (n.d.). Embracing grief: Surrendering to your sorrow has the power to heal the deepest of wounds. Sobunfu Some. www.sobonfu.com/articles/writings-by-sobonfu-2/embracing-grief

Walker, A. (2013). *Hard Times Require Furious Dancing: New Poems*. San Francisco: New World Library.

YJ Editors (2014). The yoga sequence for a healing heart. Yoga Journal, October 10. www.yogajournal.com/practice/yoga-sequences/yoga-sequence-healing-heart

PART TWO

WINTER

In Stillness

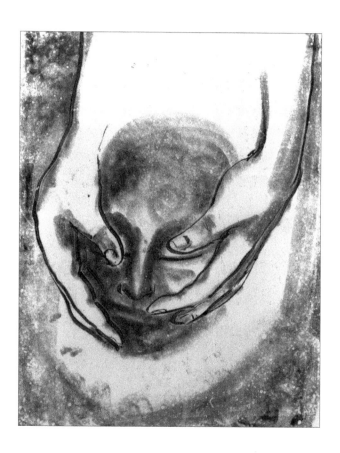

First Snow

How strange to hear the
sky cry crystal tears.
They shatter like sad
diamonds on the roof.

All evening long
it has been like this:
the whole town a snow-globe,
shaken and settling,
inexhaustible in its sudden whiteness.

Now, in the frozen
night, Earth has
covered herself with a
bleached mantle, a
silver shroud,
quiet beyond dreams.

The jealous sky too has turned
white as milk,
its luminous porcelain
fractured by the black cracks
of leafless trees.

And so we hunker down.

Even the mute beasts
know they are not
wanted out of doors.
Our dog stops short at
the threshold
    as if to ask
what icy hand
erased the world
we knew.

~ Robert A. Neimeyer

Winter Reflection

Claudia Coenen

Outside my window is a large maple, its branches spreading parallel to the ground, a knot like a small doorway into the depths on its trunk. I gaze at this knot, imagine entering the interior of the tree, which transforms into a dark tunnel. Darkness embraces me as I descend; fear tingles along the edges of the unknown.

The tunnel opens to a sea, spreading out into the distance. Now I am floating on this black, roiling sea amidst all the shattered pieces of myself. I cast a net and gather them together, and plunge into the depths, dragging that net down with me. I am terrified that I might drown, but then I remember. I know how to swim.

Down and down, I tumble, dragging the net filled with the parts of me caught inside. At the bottom is a dark green land, with air to breathe. Soft breezes caress my skin, the net rests nearby with its huge pile of jagged shards. Lying on sweetly scented grass, I rest on the ground.

There is music on the breeze, a soft humming. It is my own life, pulsing just beyond awareness, waiting to be crafted. Next to me on the shore of my own Self is the net. The shards are glittering, multi-faceted and radiantly colored. Gently, I open the net and take them out. Examining each one, I see that each is an aspect of who I am. Each fragment has something to tell.

I pick up a random piece of myself. It is an iridescent blue. It is my creativity, inspiring me to express my feelings in movement and shape. Holding it in my hand, I rise and dance on the shore of my broken self. My dance expresses the hope of healing, and as I move, I sense that I will be able to heal.

Here is a big chunk, upside down so all I see is a rough, cracked surface. This is me, the wife. I pick up this piece and it shatters into a million pieces which blow away into the breeze. I am no longer a wife now that he is dead. A huge part of my identity is gone. I fold into myself, bring my knees to my chest, sobbing. He is dead, I feel dead; how can I go on? Slowly, as my tears subside, I realize that I am not just a wife or a widow. I am still me even though he is no longer here. I will have to develop a different kind of connection with him as I rebuild my own life. One of the shattered pieces flutters by, his face smiling at me on its shining surface.

A chill wind blows, whipping my hair into my eyes. I feel a rush of memory and see him standing on a hill. He is slowly walking, observant, pausing to look at the sky, taking a drag on his cigarette. Stooping down, he touches the stalks of herbs that have died back. He straightens up and walks, slowly fading away.

I know that seeds of growth are stirring, deep beneath the frozen earth of winter. In the dark, we incubate the possibilities of living again. Swathed in blankets by a fire, soft music playing in the background to soothe our troubles, we slow down. Snow falls, changing the landscape and hiding what has died. Deep in our hearts, we know that grief cannot really hide; it exists alongside love and longing.

CHAPTER 6

Crossing the Threshold of Embodiment and Imagination

Evie Lindemann

"Art, when inspired with love, leads to higher realms. Love art, and that art will open for you the inner life."

Meher Baba (Purdom, 1937)

Life and death are embedded into the human experience, sometimes right in front of us, and sometimes far behind us, like a shadow. It is an ever-present reality, one which challenges us to reflect upon our own mortality, and the possibility of losing those we hold most dear. In the words of Frank Ostaseki (2017):

> Death is not waiting for us at the end of a long road. Death is always with us, in the marrow of every passing moment. She is the secret teacher hiding in plain sight, helping us to discover what matters most.

Recently, on a trip to Ireland to uncover some of my Irish roots, I stood on top of an ancient burial mound, some 220 feet in diameter, in a valley adjacent to the River Boyne. I climbed up 40 feet to get to the top, and from there I saw 17 smaller burial mounds nearby and a valley rich with patches of dazzling green fields. The base of the mound was encircled by very large stones, called kerbstones, whose surfaces contained carved spirals, diamond shapes, and serpentine forms. In amazement, I wondered about the meaning of this monument, built 5000 years ago. It made me realize that far back in our ancestral roots, these complex architectural structures, older than Stonehenge and the pyramids of Giza, were built to house the dead. Surely, the fact that this was in the Celtic culture that far back in time, with the idea of honoring the remains of the dead and burying them with small artifacts, meant the passage from life into death carried great significance. These sites, and other similar ones, were apparently places of worship, ritual, communal gathering, and remembering the ancestors.

Thomas Laqueur (2015) reminds us that no culture in the world is indifferent to human remains, and that, psychologically and emotionally, we have a need to establish continuing relationships with the dead. The physical remains of those we have loved offer a way to invest in and maintain enduring connections. In this respect, the dead help the living to connect the past and the future, and to keep culture alive through memory. While death severs our physical connections with those we love, the complex task of remembering them and learning to live without them offers the possibility of discovering ways to place those we have lost into an alternate space, as they did in the Boyne Valley. Using the expressive therapies can assist in the task of symbolically restoring to us those whom we have lost and discovering new ways to maintain connection. These therapies may include one or more of the following: visual art making, writing and poetry, movement and dance, music, and drama. In the grief work of William Worden (2009), we are reminded that the fourth task of grieving is to find an enduring connection with the deceased.

Using the expressive therapies can assist in the task of symbolically restoring to us those whom we have lost and discovering new ways to maintain connection.

I considered some of my own personal losses, and how I used art making and visual journaling to find a way through grief. I am reminded of the explorations of Stephen Levine (2019), who writes about the method of poiesis, in which difficulty is engaged by letting go of forcing an outcome and softening into the use of the imagination. What emerges is attention paid in the moment to whatever arises. The practice requires this sequence: understanding the initial therapeutic situation, a movement away from the situation and into the realm of the imagination, the creating and making of an object, spending active time with the image, and, in the return, to build a bridge between the object itself and the client's life situation.

Some years ago, during a particularly arid time in my life, the netted fabric securing the bottom of an antique chair became loosened. With half of the dusty netting touching the floor, I ripped it from underneath the chair on an impulse guided by frustration. My first thought was to toss it into a recycle bin. However, even with decades of dust attached to the filaments, my fingers began a spontaneous dance of engagement with the fabric, leading me to the sink rather than the recycle bin. As tap water seeped into the material, it became heavier in my hands and the water falling to the bottom of the sink became saturated with gray-brown dirt. I rinsed the fabric repeatedly. With each washing, the fabric became lighter in color, nearly white, until no more pools of dirty water remained. I squeezed the excess water from the fabric delicately and stretched it out on a dry towel, smoothing away the wrinkles. As I gazed at it, pocked with unusual holes from the nails that had held it in place for so many decades, I fell in love with this old piece of cloth. My artistic imagination had been awakened.

This love story wove its way into a new print, unlike any I had made previously. I inked up the torn fabric with oil-based ink and a brayer, and ran it through the press on a piece of black printmaking paper. When I removed the cloth from the paper at the far end of the press bed, I gasped at the beauty and intricacy that this worn piece of cloth had left on the paper. The story of its life and its functionality now remained through its permanent markings on the black textured surface, its voice and its messages emerging from the shadowy darkness. The places where the nails had torn the fabric remained as organically shaped holes in the image, with the black background emerging as another part of its story. Foreground and background began to interact. Continuing with the beginnings of this new print process, I studied these holes and decided that they merited expansion via an enlargement 20 times greater than their original size. In short order, I took these newly emergent shapes and created a transfer onto the finest, most transparent Japanese paper I could find.

These enlarged shapes left another story, this one of curving arches, blobs, and radiating spirals that seemed to suggest an ancient garment. I attached them to the black paper with archival glue, superimposing them over the netted pattern of the fabric. Perhaps it was becoming a brown robed monk. Perhaps, instead, it represented an abstract swirling cosmic pattern. I spent several weeks staring at this image that contained proportions of both regular and exaggerated sizes, wondering what it needed. Finally, in desperation, I spoke directly to the print, inquiring about its needs. It communicated back to me: "I need a face," and the face emerged from a central section shaped like a teardrop. First, the mouth, then the nose, and finally the eyes came into focus. Who was this person? I had no idea. In some moment of lucidity inspired by my pen and my writing paper, I asked the image to tell me about itself, and I made a commitment to listen to its answer and make use of the answer in my art. My questions covered the basics: "Who are you, where are you from, what is your name?" I wrote down what it communicated to me, but I was unprepared for its answers. The image informed me that it was St. Jerome, situated in the desert. Besides not knowing who this St. Jerome was, I also wondered why he was passing his time in the desert. In honoring my agreement to write down, listen, and make use of what was shared, I titled the piece "St. Jerome in the Desert."

Still very mystified, I did a search about St. Jerome. As it turns out, he was an historic figure who spent some years cleaning up his psyche and his personal life by leaving the city and living a life of reflection in the desert. He became a Doctor of the Early Church and was the first scholar to translate the Hebrew Bible into Latin. He often meditated on a skull, thus reminding himself of his mortality and his search for purpose. During one deeply meditative session, he was told that he needed to turn his attention away from secular writing and direct his talents to spiritual themes.

Later, I discovered multiple paintings from the Renaissance depicting St. Jerome. Legend has it that he was befriended by a lion, whose paw was swollen from a thorn embedded into its flesh. With a deft touch, St. Jerome removed it, and the two of them forged a lasting friendship.

The lion is depicted in those paintings as well, a kind of protector from the natural world, looking out for his companion. After discovering this history, I completed a second piece of art, a collage that included the figure of St. Jerome, his lion companion, and the skull in a desert setting. While my first piece was a close-up of St. Jerome, the second one included him in the larger context of his life circumstances and physical environment. The close-up gaze and the more distanced gaze are both part of the healing process of resolving grief. Symbolically, we must enter into the image itself in a direct and emotional way, and then step back to view it in a larger context. It brings the realms of feeling and cognition together.

In a parallel process, I began to understand why St. Jerome had entered the field of my artistic imagination. We had many things in common. I had lived in a desert of sorts in my personal life for five years, following the extended illness and deaths of my sister, then my mother, and the ending of my marriage. This season of my life was as dry as a desert, and I had a great deal of time to contemplate and experience loss, endings, emotional challenges, and deeper questions about the quality of my life, my relationships, and my mortality. The meanings that had previously given my life dignity no longer fit, just as the meanings that St. Jerome had held dear no longer fit into his landscape. I was forced to begin again by entering what I would later describe as the underworld.

This region is shadowed, dark, mysterious, frightening, and lonely. I knew that my healing depended upon my willingness to say yes to this descent, and I did. I listened in earnest for inspiration, for guidance, for an opening in my heart. Very slowly, as the arid, heavy quality of my emotional desert began to lift, St. Jerome found me through my printmaking, reminding me of the seasons of life and of a reawakening of the embodied spiritual values and teachings that I hold dear. When I say that St. Jerome found me, I know that my artistic imagination is a mystery, and I never really understand from whence arise my ideas and imagery. Rather than being the director of the imagery, I feel instead that I am the conduit for the mystery and beauty of creative possibilities. And so it was that St. Jerome found me. This approach is in keeping with the practice of poiesis.

I tell this story to illustrate how it is that my art imagery parallels my life experiences, and how it is that I consider mark making and personal reflection as sacred acts that facilitate psychic and spiritual integration. When a person can consciously be engaged with her or his art by being willing to simply listen and follow imaginative travels, art creates a pathway into the rich environment of an inner life. Following an integrative process permits me to cross the threshold into a different realm of experience, a healing sanctuary. From these crossings, my understanding deepens, enriches, mystifies, enchants, and informs me.

In 2007, years before St. Jerome made his way into my artistic imagination, I began teaching art therapy to graduate students. I undertook a study of Jung's practice of engaging his patients in expressive directions, such as painting, dancing, and writing. He called this method "active imagination" (Chodorow, 1997), in which he encouraged his patients to interact directly with their imagery by writing about it, developing dialogues, and dancing the images into three-dimensional being. Jung believed that active imagination facilitated the building of a bridge between their creative expressions and their internal lives. This was not an intellectual exercise, but rather a direct engagement with their inner lives via their art creations. This form of excavative work permitted them to explore their personal associations to their images, and later to amplify the process by finding out about the lore and mythological features potentially connected to their particular symbolism.

The active imagination process, and other processes that have been developed from Jung's original pattern, broadened the playing field of artistic products in therapy, removing them from a strictly product-oriented approach with a fixed analytical position. Rather, both the process of creation and a finished product offer a great gift in therapy. It signals a coming to know oneself in an original way, opening a door to an experiential exploration of one's struggles, conflicts, and triumphs from a more deeply embedded location in the psyche. Art processes and products become aspects of an enlivened journey rather than a procedure with a definitive ending. Art becomes a way station on the pilgrimage of inner knowing, as exemplified by the quote with which this chapter began. The willingness to engage in a process in which control of outcomes is surrendered and the individual is open and available to not knowing can lead to a powerful aesthetic response that is, in itself, a change agent with deep meaning.

Since the development of Jung's active imagination process, many other approaches to the inner and outer world of imagination and creativity have been developed. For example, current practice in the field of art therapy includes the use of both created artwork and visual journaling as a field of reflective inquiry for graduate interns learning the therapeutic uses of art with clients. Visual journaling involves both creating art imagery as well as writing about it. It is this process that led St. Jerome to my printmaking practice. I have used this inner/outer practice for years, which allows me to "peek" behind my images and discover their symbolic underpinnings and the inner work this artwork either suggests or requires of me.

I like to start my visual journaling process with an embodied beginning of yogic breathing practices that help to focus my mind, calm my nervous system, and create a spacious integration of bodily processes, feeling states, and thought processes. From this "ground of being," sensations arise, as do smells, sights, sounds, and textures, all of which become part of the art-making process. This may well be the sixth sense of imagination, the realm in which duality is softened, and the place where a state of connection and integration occurs. This work can be extremely subtle, suggesting a liminal experience, a space "in between," in which some of the deeper realities in the psyche are uncovered and revealed. It requires paying careful attention in each moment, enlivening the present with a quivering sense of aliveness and fullness. The spaciousness of this engagement leads me to new image making on paper, within a large black spiral-bound, unlined art book. The fact that the emerging images are contained within the covers of the black book provides a sense of safety in those moments when what arises may shift from lovely to frightening. Following the development of a visual image, I pick up my pen and allow the image to "speak" to me in the language of "I." An example of how this works is the following dialogue from one of my etchings. A central figure in the image had this to say:

> I am a woman looking ahead rather than back. The moon is rising. I am bathed in moonlight and I sense the rhythm of the moon and tides, of the darkening evening, of the quiet around me. I am guided by my capacity to be with these forces of nature. My heart is calm, I am at peace with the mysteries.

In the lower left corner of this same image, a smaller figure spoke. She said:

> I gaze into the unknown and the unknowable. I offer you a doorway, and I tell you to come this way, to come through the portal, to cross the threshold. It will be all right. You are ready.

This interactive flow between the art maker and the image offers a rich field for play, for learning, and for enhanced creativity. Rollo May described a particular occurrence in the life of creative individuals that he called the encounter (May, 1975). May believed that in order to pave the way for this kind of creative encounter, a period of solitude and quiet reflection was required. During this experience, the usual conflicts and polarizations that occur in daily living cease for the moment, and during this time, something rises up from the unconscious and erupts into awareness. When a break-through occurs, it creates a disruption in currently held beliefs, and may, in fact, destroy preciously held paradigms that one held dear. The disruption of former beliefs and ideas is an act of destruction, ironically occurring in the wake of a creative emergence, which is similar to Picasso's view that "Every act of creation is first an act of destruction." May also proposed that this experience facilitates a kind of clarity and vividness in the moment of breakthrough, and that it only occurs when the person is completely com-mitted to the problem at hand. The intentionality of process described by

May reflects the same kind of focused awareness and attention described earlier in the visual journaling approach. Visual journaling is a similar process in that it encompasses May's ideas about "the encounter," provides a space for quietude and reflection, for active art making, and for a way into the significance of the imagery through writing about it. The special gifts embodied by art making offer a way to follow a process, create artwork, and unwrap imaginative and creative discoveries that move in the direction of an enhancement of the inner life.

When individuals choose to interact with their art in this way, they often end up with not only a title for their artwork but also a description of what the art embodies for them. This crossing of the threshold, from creating the artwork itself and then engaging with it in an embodied way, completes the creative cycle. It can, for example, be a wonderful addition to an art show when an artist offers more than a title for appreciating her or his work and includes some of the symbolic inner process and meaning of the art making. This addition becomes an invitation to viewers to travel into the work they are viewing by doing some of their own corresponding inner work.

At the same time, in the therapeutic realm, the practice of combining visual journaling in working with clients who are experiencing grief and loss holds great promise. After creating an image, the writing process helps to ground and contain the experience, offering both an aesthetic distance as well as potential deep insight. Remembering the idea of poiesis, when therapist and client are able to meet in the liminal space of not knowing, of being in the present moment, an energy exchange occurs, one that offers both individuals the opportunity to join in a way that diminishes a sense of isolation and loss that is so common in the experience of grief. It also creates an environment in which the client experiences a kind of freedom to take risks and to begin to explore the sources of their grief through the power of the imagination.

References

Chodorow, J. (1997). *Jung on Active Imagination*. Princeton, NJ: Princeton University Press.

Laqueur, T. (2015). *The Work of the Dead: A Cultural History of Mortal Remains*. Princeton, NJ: Princeton University Press.

Levine, S.K. (2019). *Philosophy of Expressive Arts Therapy: Poiesis and the Therapeutic Imagination*. London and Philadelphia, PA: Jessica Kingsley Publishers.

May, R. (1975). *The Courage to Create*. New York: Norton & Co.

Ostaseki, F. (2017). *The Five Invitations: Discovering What Death Can Teach Us About Living Fully*. New York, NY: Flatiron Books.

Purdom, C.B. (1937). *The Perfect Master*. London: Williams & Norgate.

Worden, W.J. (2009). *Counselling and Grief Therapy: A Handbook for the Mental Health Practitioner*. New York, NY: Routledge.

CHAPTER 7

Journaling Through Grief and Beyond

Heather Stang

I was introduced to journaling in ninth-grade English class. My cohort and I were required to write three pages in a spiral-bound notebook every night for the term. The teacher did not collect our journals but viewed them from a respectable distance, ensuring our homework was complete without invading our privacy.

This practice was transformational. Even though my words were not intended for an audience, the thoughts in my head mirrored on the thin blue lines made me feel witnessed, validated, and somehow more in control.

Eventually, I decided to share the feelings I was processing with my teacher after class while building a replica Globe Theater for a Shakespeare project. I found I had more clarity around what was bothering me about life.

The themes in that first journal contained what you would expect from any adolescent. Boredom in school, frustration with my parents, gossip about friends, unrequited love, and what I imagined my adult life would be like.

But what impacted me the most then, and still does to this day, were the entries about my mother's brother—Uncle Doug—who died by suicide when I was seven. I didn't know it then, but my teacher inspired my first grief journal.

In that red spiral-bound notebook, I recalled the time he took me to see the just-released *Snow White* movie in the Raleigh Theater. Afterward, we went to a record store—no doubt one he frequented often—where he bought the Disney soundtrack and a blue plastic ring from a gumball machine for me. I never intentionally got rid of that ring, but it has since disappeared. Sometimes I dig through my jewelry box, looking for it. I wrote him letters asking why he did what he did and letting him know I still loved him.

My journal did not judge me when I confessed that I rummaged through my grandmother's files in the middle of the night to find a disappointingly brief police report from a small town in Alaska that revealed a secret my grandmother had been keeping from all of us: the cocaine residue on the handgun found at the scene. I didn't share that knowledge with anyone until over three decades later when my grandmother was too far gone to confront.

It gave me a safe place to vent my anger at anyone who damned people like my uncle to hell, question if my religious views were really mine, and wonder if I would live past 26—something Dougy did not.

I also recorded what I now know as the beginning of the end of my parents' union, processing the heartbreaking loss of trust I had for my father specifically and marriage in general. Soon after this entry, he "found" my secret reflections. After a screaming match, he confiscated the journal, never to be seen again.

I feel like my adolescent grieving process was interrupted by this violation. To this day, I mourn the loss of this artifact. How I would love to read those thoughts now that I am an adult, not to mention a grief professional.

But all is not lost. I feel in my heart and bones that the practice of writing was not in vain. I recall the original events in the 1970s, *and* the act of writing them down in the 1980s, *and* the many times I revisited these themes over the years. Each time, I learn something different about my love, loss, and constantly changing self.

Free Writing to Let It All Out

There are many styles of journaling. Free writing, also known as stream of consciousness, is the style of writing most associated with keeping a journal and what I learned in high school. This is simply writing down whatever is on your mind, moving your hand continuously as you write or type—even if you write the same phrase over and over again: "I don't know what to write. I don't know what to write. I don't know what to write."

All the rules get tossed out the window. Proper spelling, grammar, punctuation, and even page margins are sacrificed for raw, unfiltered emotion. You do not need to make sense, write in a linear fashion, or tie the story up in a neat little bow.

It is important for me not to be precious about what I write. I'm a writer by trade, but content and grammar don't matter in my journal. Angry scribbles are just as valuable as poetic images. (Rebecca F.)

Free writing can release deeply held beliefs and insights that were previously obscured. I find that once I get my conscious thoughts on paper, the juicy stuff starts to come out. This is why it is important to write nonstop and without judgment. Of course, we all encounter our inner critic (I am struggling with mine now). But remember that you are not sharing your journal with anyone and are free to say whatever you need to.

One thing to consider is whether to be traditional and use a pen and paper or go digital. Paper allows you to unplug and free yourself from digital distractions, and blank pages create space to express yourself freely. Paper journals are also portable, so you can write wherever you are comfortable and experiment with writing in different settings, such as outdoors or in a coffee shop. The flexibility of paper means you can write down your interior flow of thoughts and observations without limits.

I combine writing with drawing pictures and incorporating color. It's important for me to choose the right journal. I like something unlined so that I can write, draw, and color at will. It needs to be spiral-bound so it can lie flat on the desk and large enough so I don't feel cramped. Getting the right tools for journaling, including some beautiful pens, feels like an act of self-love. (Rebecca F.)

Because writing on paper is slower than typing, you become more intimate with your narrative and are more likely to gain insight. Here are some things to consider:

- What is the ideal size for you?
- Do you prefer lined, grid, or unlined paper?
- Spiral- or perfect-bound?
- Simple or fancy cover?
- What paper texture appeals to you?
- What pens or pencils will you most enjoy using?

If you will collage or use paint pens that might bleed through the paper, find an art sketchbook with heavier-weight paper.

The downside to paper is that anyone can read it (as I learned firsthand), so be sure to store it in a safe place. Digital options are easy to secure, and if you do not like to write by hand, they offer the luxury of typing or dictation. Be mindful that the increased speed doesn't prevent you from savoring rich subject matter. Whether you use a computer or smartphone, a text document, or an online journaling platform (such as 750 Words or AfterTalk), bring the same mindfulness to your breath and body just as you would when writing by hand, and savor rich content.

As Natalie Goldberg shares in *Writing Down the Bones* (2016), "Lose control. Don't think. Don't get logical. Go for the jugular. (If something comes up in your writing that is scary or naked, dive right into it. It probably has lots of energy.)"

Guided Journals to Expand Your Narrative

While writing with wild abandon can help you process and release pent-up emotions, if you start to feel that your journal is just another space for constant worry and rumination, or feel bored or retraumatized when you write, guided journals and writing prompts can help you get unstuck.

> When my husband died, I kept a journal. I was so angry, because it was so unfair, the way he died. I know I needed to get that out—it was like the anger was stuck in me and had to get out. But repeating the same story over and over made me angrier. I was convinced journaling didn't work for me, so I gave up. Then I heard about guided journals in my grief group. I got a few different kinds, one for widows and *From Grief to Peace*. Even though it seemed crazy at the time, I got one on gratitude. I go back and forth between them, depending on what I feel I need in the moment. They all help, and now if I write in my old journal, I have more to say. I'm still angry. It still isn't fair. But now I write about other feelings too. Like how much I miss him. How much I still love him. (Keisha B.)

Writing prompts are not only the antidote to writer's block and rumination; responding to specific types of questions can help improve prolonged grief disorder, depressive, and post-traumatic stress symptoms, as well as physical health. A study by Lichtenthal and Cruess (2010) compared traditional "non-directed emotional disclosure" with directed writing that focused on two elements of post-loss meaning making: sense making and benefit finding.

The traditional group wrote about their "deepest thoughts and emotions related to their loss." The sense-making group wrote about what they felt caused the death and how the experience changed their life, close relationships, and worldview. The benefit-finding group reflected on any positive life changes that are a result of their loss experience. A fourth group objectively described the room in which they were seated.

Of the four groups, those focused on meaning making were more effective than writing about neutral topics. Emotional disclosure had some benefits, though not as much as the meaning-making prompts.

I am grateful for this study. Not only does it give grief professionals insight into what works, but it is what prompted my publisher to reach out and ask me to write a guided journal based on my first book, *Mindfulness and Grief* (Stang, 2024). The result is *From Grief to Peace* (Stang, 2021). Both of these books follow an eight-step process I developed that tends first to the emotional overwhelm and physical symptoms of grief, then moves the client gently forward towards meaning making and post-traumatic growth. This system is also described in "Mindfulness-based Grief Therapy," a chapter in the *Handbook of Grief Therapies* (Steffen, Milman, & Neimeyer, 2023).

Writing prompts can be found on the internet, or you can make up your own. Just ask yourself a question and write out the answer. Guided journals are a collection of writing prompts. Some of them have the same material on every page, while others are designed to move you in a direction or give variety.

Your local bookseller will have good suggestions. If you purchase one online, be sure to verify that the book you buy includes prompts. There are many blank journals that appear to be guided because of the cover design.

Guided Writing Prompt

The thing I am most proud of about myself since the loss is _____.

(From Grief to Peace, *Stang, 2021, p.121)*

Gratitude for What Is Left

Although I don't view grief as a gift, I am grateful for the love, support, and comfort I received from friends, families, and even strangers during difficult times. Turning toward the good when you are writing can help balance your mood, reduce anxiety, and make you feel less alone. Like other writing prompts, focusing on gratitude expands your awareness and helps you get unstuck. As Kristin Armstrong, author and ex-wife of Lance Armstrong, writes, "When we focus on our gratitude, the tide of disappointment goes out and the tide of love rushes in" (2008).

Like all practices, gratitude should never be forced or used as a spiritual bypass. There is a right timing to this feeling, and if you aren't ready, that just means you aren't ready.

You can purchase guided gratitude journals or simply keep a list of three things you were grateful for that day. The impact is far greater, however, if you spend time really savoring one to three things that you appreciate. Bring your body into it, cultivating a sense of appreciation, and let those feelings out onto the page.

Guided Writing Prompt

Today I am most grateful for _____ because _____.

Art Journals

Sometimes there are no words to express how you feel. Sketches, paint, found objects, colors, photographs, collages, and natural items can be as powerful as writing. Even if you find writing helpful, incorporating visual elements into your grief journal offers a new way of "seeing" what you feel inside.

The first art journal I saw belonged to a widow participating in a grief group at my meditation center. All sorts of media spilled over the edges of her hard-backed book. Fabric, leaves, watercolors, cutouts from magazines, copies of treasured photographs, and written reflections recorded whatever she felt in the moment without any limits. Her journal overflowed with feelings, memories, wisdom, and her authentic expression of anger, sadness, love, and hope.

You do not need to be an artist to create an art journal. If you find drawing intimidating as I do, use crayons! They hold no expectation of artistic acumen. Or find a pair of scissors and a glue stick; then cut out whatever moves you from magazines or printouts from the internet.

Guided Art Exercise

Take a walk outside and pay attention to what you see, including the sky, earth, plants, animals, and signs of weather. Then, using crayons or collage, create a landscape that is a metaphor for your grief. Is it day or night? Are you in the ocean, a desert, a city, or wilderness? Perhaps your grief feels like another planet. Use the traditional landscape elements as a starting point, but don't feel limited by them (Stang, 2024, p.90).

Warming Up and Getting Unstuck

Anyone who has ever had to write anything knows how intimidating a blank page can be. Whether you are paralyzed by writer's block, wrestling your inner critic, or struggling with anxiety or deep sadness, here are a few tips to help move you forward.

One way to get unstuck is to move your body. Many people find that a walk or yoga before journaling clears away the mental chatter that can get in the way of a fluid journaling session. It can help release anxious energy and help focus your mind.

You can also get into the flow by warming up your writing muscles before diving into the juicy stuff. Set a timer for between one and five minutes and write about something that isn't ripe with emotion. Describe an object on your desk. Make a daily "to-do" list that is taking up space in your mind. Search for "photo of the day" on the internet and describe what you see in detail.

Once you start journaling for grief, you may discover that you write about the same thing over and over again. This is a normal part of processing your loss. In addition to guided journals and writing prompts, creative narrative techniques can help you explore your story in a new way:

- Write with your nondominant hand.
- Switch your point of view from the first person to third (or even second).
- Craft a dialogue between two or more people using different color pens for each person.
- Explore descriptive details as specifically as possible, down to the minutia.
- Draw or collage a storyboard scene by scene as if outlining a movie.
- Intentionally misspell words and ignore grammar rules.
- Rotate your journal 90 degrees or completely upside down.

Guided Writing Warm-Up

- One minute: Pick out one physical object in the room and describe it without emotion (objective).
- Three minutes: Write what you like most about a book, TV show, or movie (opinion).
- Five minutes: Find the strongest sensation in your body and compare it to a weather event (comparison).

Time to Write

Many people generally resist journaling and self-care practices because they believe they don't have the time. While I am not here to dispute anyone's level of busyness, I think there is a belief that journaling is the same as writing an essay for school or a proposal for work. Thank goodness this is not the case!

The key is to create a sustainable practice that works for you. Maybe it is five minutes of free writing after coffee in the morning. Maybe you shut the office door and fill three lined pages at lunch, or spend 15 minutes following the prompts in your guided journal at night.

We can toss out time goals completely and commit that pen will touch paper once a day, if only to write, "I showed up. That is enough for today."

That being said, I do believe that a regular writing practice is most helpful. I also believe that if you are free-writing, it can take some time to declutter the conscious mind.

But as with meditation, frequency is more important than duration. As with any healing practice, journaling shouldn't cause extra suffering. Whether you write for one minute or one hour, it is time well spent.

Benefits of Journaling Through Grief (and Beyond)

Unleash Your Authentic Self

Pent-up emotions can act like a volcano raging inside. Stuff your feelings long enough and you may notice they start to leak out in small but hurtful jabs or erupt in a devastating outburst. Emotion regulation can help you and those around you live a more peaceful life, but it is important to balance that with an authentic relationship with yourself.

Journaling releases the pressure in a private, contained space, so you can untangle and process your feelings on your own terms without judgment or negative consequences. It is a relief to relinquish dark or taboo feelings to the page, like flushing toxins out of your system. This is not to minimize the hurt, pain, anger, or whatever you are feeling, but is designed to relieve the pressure and make space for you to *tend* to the feeling rather than *react* to it.

In *Lessons of Loss* (2000), Dr. Robert Neimeyer shares, "Especially when losses are traumatic, they may be difficult to discuss or even disclose to another. And yet the psychological and physical burden of harboring painful memories without the release of sharing can prove far more destructive in the long run."

> I turned to journaling right away after the sudden loss of my husband. It helped me feel and share the unimaginable pain that instantly dominated my life. I am learning you have to feel the pain of loss before you can get through it. And journaling allows me to share my thoughts, emotions, and grief with someone I could trust. Myself. It helped me to trust myself. (Bushia, private correspondence)

Pent-up emotions can act like a volcano raging inside. Stuff your feelings long enough and you may notice they start to leak out in small but hurtful jabs or erupt in a devastating outburst. Emotion regulation can help you and those around you live a more peaceful life, but it is important to balance that with an authentic relationship with yourself.

One of the kindest things you can do for yourself through grief is to treat yourself just as you would treat a beloved friend in the same circumstance. Start by being radically honest with yourself in the privacy of your grief journal. You may uncover thoughts and feelings you didn't even know you had.

Journaling has been one of the most helpful tools for me in living through grief. I process the events of my life by writing them down, and I'm often surprised to look back over what I've written and see how my emotions are revealed to me on the page. (Rebecca F., private correspondence)

Don't hold back. Don't pretend everything is OK when it isn't. Don't censor yourself to protect other people's feelings. Release your anger, regret, fear, rage, jealousy, betrayal, despair, relief, and everything else you are afraid to admit out loud onto the page. Your journal can handle it.

Guided Writing Prompt

What I really want those who care about me to know is _____.

(From Grief to Peace, *Stang, 2021, p.65)*

Savor the Memories

Memory is a quirky thing. Sometimes we forget what we want to remember; other times we remember what we want to forget. Over time, telling your story of love and loss may leave you struggling to recall the elusive details: the timeframe of the diagnosis ("Was it the 26th or 28th?"), who said what to whom ("I think it was Aunt Barb—no, it was definitely Norine"). Even details that at the time felt larger than life start to diminish.

Some details matter, others less so. But if you know you want to always remember something, write it down. Thirteen years after my stepfather died from a pulmonary embolism after coming home from surgery, I still struggle to remember what he had me pick up for lunch. I know I bought cheeseburgers, French fries, and milkshakes, but was it three or four of each? The importance of detail is in the eye of the beholder. No one else cares how many calories I purchased that day, but I sure do. (I think it was three. No, four. See what I mean?)

Journaling helps your brain commit an event to memory and process its impact, and this is especially true when writing by hand. It makes more of an impact in your memory center and creates a written record that you can revisit anytime.

Whether or not you come back to a journal entry is your choice. Some people find it very therapeutic to reread their own words, even when the memory is painful. Your own words validate your experience and may offer a new perspective.

You can also journal as a way to share memories with other loved ones, like children who are too small to remember:

I keep a journal primarily to communicate with my daughter, Khloey, who was only two and a half when her father, Mike, died. Writing down answers to her questions and memories helps me know what I want to share. The other day, I asked her if she remembered him, and, of course, she said, "No." I told her, "Well, you are going to remember him through me. What I write, the pictures, photos, his best friends telling stories—that is how you are going to know who he is. You will know that he loved you." He used to say he loved us so much it felt like Disney Magic. I am printing out all of the social media posts he made about her from the day I said "I think I am pregnant" to when we brought her home and beyond. (KaySea, personal correspondence)

Guided Writing Prompt

1. For five minutes, make a list of everything you want to always remember.
2. Choose one item from your list and write about it in your journal for at least 15 minutes, savoring as many details as you can remember.
3. Add to this list anytime you remember something and continue to use the list for individual writing prompts.

Nurture the Love That Remains

Journaling for me consists of a continuing letter to my departed wife about what I'm doing and thinking. One might consider this a one-way conversation, but after 63 years of marriage, I can hear her responding to my musings. So she is still helping me stay grounded, centered, and patient as I deal with my grief and move to my new normal. (Joshua, private correspondence)

My stepfather, Tom Clark, was the son of a *Life Magazine* photographer best known for images of Marilyn Monroe and the Kennedy's Camelot era that graced the covers and pages of the magazine and monographs alike. Tom carried on the family tradition by photographing lavish embassy parties for the *Washington Post* and eventually opened a studio specializing in family photos, business headshots, photo restoration, and 24-hour film development.

I wasn't allowed to touch my stepfather's camera when he was alive. It took me four months after he died to get the courage to pick it up. Even then, I was certain I would be struck by lightning. I survived, and, not too long after, wrote him a letter explaining that I would take care of his camera, and how each time I looked through a lens, it made me feel like I was seeing through his eyes.

I also penned a response from him, which gave me the permission I craved along with encouragement for my newfound hobby. While the letter I wrote in my stepfather's words emerged organically, a number of grief and writing professionals encourage this type of back-and-forth communication (Kennedy, 2009; Neimeyer, 2012).

What a relief this is to so many who wonder if they are out of their mind for not only talking to their loved one but feeling a sense of comfort from doing so. Maintaining what Klass, Silverman, and Nickman (1996) called the *continuing bond* is so normal that many of us do it without even knowing it has a name.

Letter writing can help us acknowledge and tend to our deep yearning for our loved one's presence. While some will feel ready to write to their loved one right away, in my experience, many bereaved people begin letter writing after the acute symptoms of grief have started to settle. The journal begins to transform from a coping tool into a vessel of meaning making and continuing connection:

> After 18 months on this journey, I have recently changed how I journal. Until now, I would journal any time the need struck, which was any time of day. Maybe the middle of the night. But now, I save journaling time for the last thing I do before my head hits the pillow. And I am writing directly to my husband. You see, I've recently felt him very much a part of life as before but in a very different form. A spiritual form. Writing to him every night has helped me feel that I am directly talking to him. I am feeling and sharing with the one other person in my life that I trust—many times more than I trust myself. It helps me feel closer to him. And support from him as I know he would give it. (Bushia)

This practice is not limited to healthy relationships, though self-compassion and emotional safety should always be front of mind when writing to or from a difficult or abusive person. In her book *The Infinite Thread* (2009, p.72), Alexandra Kennedy advises:

> You may need to express uncomfortable feelings, thoughts, and memories before you can move on to feeling compassionate, loving, or understanding. And it may take several letters to get to a point of closure...you can actively participate in this process, but you can't control or force it.

My interpretation of "closure" in this passage isn't that everything will feel as though it is wrapped up in a nice, neat bow, all harm erased, but that you have done what you can *for yourself* to tend to the suffering that you are carrying. This may be writing the response to your letter in an idealized tone so you can hear the words you need to hear or writing in their actual tone so you can see the truth of their behavior. How you choose to do this can be informed by your needs and beliefs surrounding what happens after death.

My relationship with my stepfather wasn't always easy. There were some very dark periods where he skipped his medication for bipolar disorder and engaged in reckless behavior that had a long-term impact on our family. At his best, he was loving and generous, offering the unconditional acceptance I never felt with my birth father.

When I respond in "Tom's voice," I write as though we are our best selves. I can connect to his true essence: photographer, father figure, old hippie, teller of tall tales, historian, artist, dog dad, and someone who loved to overdo it when it came to good food.

Guided Writing Prompt

1. Spend at least ten minutes writing a letter to your person, beginning with: Dear (name), Since the last time I saw you, I have been thinking a lot about _____.

2. Spend another ten minutes (at least) writing a letter from your person: Dear (your name), I read your letter, and what really stands out to me is _____.

Document Your Post-Traumatic Growth

Most people would assume that working as a grief professional is depressing. I describe it as hopeful. While I do feel the gravity of my clients' pain and wish they did not have to be separated from those they love, this sadness is balanced with my knowledge that they will not just survive but will experience what scholars refer to as post-traumatic growth (Calhoun *et al.*, 2010). These significantly positive changes that emerge after a traumatic event—including the death of a loved one—are categorized into five domains:

- personal strength
- appreciation of life

- closer relationships with others
- new possibilities
- spiritual change.

Naturally, this is not a welcome transaction. I would gladly give back all of my growth to have my beloved family, friends, and pets back by my side forever. But given the reality of the situation, in time, most people can acknowledge ways they have changed for the good and start to answer the inevitable question, "Who am I *now*?"

Post-traumatic growth is not a process that can be rushed. It is an organic awakening that follows good grief work. I believe that practices including mindfulness, self-compassion, and connection with a like-minded community can act as a fertilizer of sorts. Like a seed sprouting beneath the soil, growth is not usually visible in the early season. But regular reflection in a grief journal will lead to a harvest of wisdom, self-awareness, and personal growth.

I help bereaved people cultivate post-traumatic growth week-by-week in my online grief support program, Awaken, using meditation, movement, journaling, and peer support, and emphasizing the importance of daily self-care. Awaken Pro helps us grief professionals practice what we preach while learning how to facilitate these healing practices with clients and groups.

Each week, we focus on a theme from the Mindfulness and Grief System, the foundation for my book *Mindfulness and Grief* (Stang, 2024), my guided journal *From Grief to Peace* (Stang, 2021), and is described in a chapter in *The Handbook of Grief Therapies* (Steffen *et al.*, 2023).

While everyone's experience of grief is unique, I do notice a few behaviors that are more common than not. Early on, it is not uncommon for a group member to share, "I just don't know how I am going to get through this." Then they learn self-care practices and coping skills and feel really supported by the group. "I've got this!" they exclaim. And then it hits. A tsunami of heartache bowls them over. "But I was doing so well."

In Buddhism, there are five hindrances to presence. The most dangerous one is doubt, which I think of as hopelessness. The antidote in the ancient teachings is to seek help from a wise teacher, ask questions, and read books. Let us not forget that a journal is a book; it doesn't have to be published to count.

When I was writing *Mindfulness and Grief* (Stang, 2024), I invited past participants of my eight-week yoga for grief program—the predecessor to Awaken—to sit down with me one-on-one and share how the experience impacted them *four years* after the last class. Most of them brought the grief journal they kept during the program to help jog their memory.

Much to my surprise, many were still writing. Even more surprising—both to me and my students—were the new insights that sprang forth from these dusty entries. What was recorded four years prior in their darkest days illuminated how far they had come in their ability to cope with pain and know they would survive, to honor their loved one who died every day while embarking on their new life, to connect deeply and fully with themselves and the other living beings in their life. Until this point, I thought my program was just helping people cope with grief in the early days. It took time and reflection to illustrate the bounty of post-traumatic growth.

This works for the writers, too. Remember that when doubt arises, if you write regularly, you likely have in your possession one of the wisest books on grief: your own grief journal.

What if your journal is filled only with hopeless entries? Then it is time to change *how* you journal and make a shift from free writing to guided prompts designed to move you forward while still honoring where you are. If you are feeling hopeless and contemplating suicide, please call the Suicide and Crisis Lifeline at 988 in the U.S. or call your local emergency room.

Guided Writing Prompt

Choose one type of post-traumatic growth that you see in yourself: personal strength, appreciation of life, closer relationships with others, new possibilities, or spiritual change. How do your thoughts, words, and deeds demonstrate this quality in you now? (From Stang, 2021, p.99.)

Introducing Journaling to Your Clients

Of course, the reality is that some people just don't want to journal. It may remind them of the dreaded research paper or feel like a waste of precious time. I can personally attest to not wanting to journal because I fear what might come out (which is the perfect time to journal!). I can find all sorts of excuses not to write.

Sadly, some people are not introduced to the practice in a way that sounds appealing: "My therapist told me I need to journal, but I hate writing. I do enough of that at work." Or they struggle with writer's block: "I tried to journal, but I just didn't know what to say." Or it is just too scary: "I am afraid if I start writing, I will just get so angry I won't be able to come back from it."

No one *has* to journal (unless it is part of your grade in English class). So, rather than "assign" journaling as "homework," inspire your clients by finding their preferences. Do they hate writing by hand? Talk about digital options. Prefer to draw rather than narrate? Perfect time for an art journal. Have a specific issue they are struggling with? Help them write their own prompt and encourage them to respond. Teach them how to listen to their body and ground themselves if they feel overwhelmed. If learning differences are present, lean into helpful technology such as dictation software.

Journaling to Integrate a Therapy Session

One way to introduce journaling is toward the end of a therapy session, but with plenty of time to write and reflect. This adds value by giving the client space to sort through their experience, recognize patterns, and pull out what they want to carry forward into their life. It also gives them a written record of their therapeutic journey for later reflection and helps commit the experience to memory by the very act of writing it down.

The method outlined below is the one I use at the end of private and group sessions. It is based on the Integration Meditation that I use as a Phoenix Rising[1] yoga therapist and was created by the founder, Michael Lee (2005).

Guided Writing Prompt
1. Think back to the beginning of our time together today and write down what you hoped to get out of our time together.
2. Replay this experience in your mind and write down anything that stands out to you. Include what you felt, heard, said, and didn't say.
3. Review your list and choose what feels most significant to you right now. Circle it, then write down why it is significant. When you are ready, share what you wrote with me.

Sometimes these first three steps are enough, especially for people new to therapy or journaling. If it feels beneficial, help your client create an action

---

1   https://pryt.com

step they can put into place before their next session, and have them record this in their journal.

Clinicians Are People, Too

When I was training to be a yoga therapist, my teacher and mentors emphasized the value of practicing yoga postures and breathing techniques regularly for oneself before ever offering them to a client. I apply this principle to everything in my toolkit, including movement, meditation, journaling, and other creative activities.

Firsthand experience with a technique helps me teach with more clarity, deepens my ability to be empathetic without being overwhelmed, and provides valuable self-care for me as a person and as a professional.

The line between personal and professional loss is very thin. Helping professionals not only carries our own losses but we are touched by our clients' stories of love and loss.

Whether you work with people navigating the end of life, comfort the bereaved, or work in any profession where you care deeply about the people you serve, my hope is you will treat yourself as you do your beloved clients. And if you love to journal, I hope you share it with as many people as it will help.

References

Armstrong, K. (2008). *Happily Ever After: Walking with Peace and Courage Through a Year of Divorce*. New York, NY: FaithWords.

Calhoun, L., Tedeschi, R., Cann, A., & Hanks, E. (2010). Positive outcomes following bereavement: Paths to posttraumatic growth. *Psychologica Belgica*, *50*(1–2), 125–143. https://doi.org/10.5334/pb-50-1-2-125

Goldberg, N. (2016). *Writing Down the Bones: Freeing the Writer Within*. Boston, MA: Shambhala Publications.

Kennedy, A. (2009). *The Infinite Thread: Healing Relationships beyond Loss*. Portland, OR: Beyond Words.

Klass, D., Silverman, P.R., & Nickman, S.L. (1996). *Continuing Bonds: New Understandings of Grief*. New York, NY: Routledge.

Lee, M. (2005). *Turn Stress into Bliss: The Proven 8-Week Program for Better Health, Relaxation, and Stress-Relief*. Minneapolis, MN: Quayside.

Lichtenthal, W.G. & Cruess, D.G. (2010). Effects of directed written disclosure on grief and distress symptoms among bereaved individuals. *Death Studies*, *34*(6), 475–499.

Neimeyer, R.A. (2000). *Lessons of Loss: A Guide to Coping*. New York, NY: McGraw-Hill.

Neimeyer, R.A. (2012). Correspondence with the Deceased. In R.A. Neimeyer (ed.) *Techniques of Grief Therapy: Creative Practices for Counseling the Bereaved*. New York, NY: Routledge.

Stang, H. (2021). *From Grief to Peace: A Guided Journal for Navigating Loss with Compassion and Mindfulness*. New York, NY: Ryland Peters & Small.

Stang, H. (2024). *Living with Grief: With Guided Meditations to Calm the Mind and Restore the Spirit* (2nd ed.). New York, NY: Ryland Peters & Small.

Steffen, E.M., Milman, E., & Neimeyer, R.A. (eds) (2023). *The Handbook of Grief Therapies*. London: Sage.

CHAPTER 8

The Cinematic Winter

Film and Working with Grief
Yon Walls

Bone Stillness

Yesterday I
had scent of you,
your warm flesh

When a daughter
I hadn't remembered it,
but now,
sensory and solid
as meeting a bare tree
in December

Being in that vividness
of moment
I knew you again,
as in that film we both loved,
you called out
to come back, smiling

and then, you vanished,
as a noble grain
of sand

The Human Experience of Grief Through Cinema

When I wrote this poem, I had finally begun to thaw from my grief. Grief is hard. Grief is transforming, can be liberating, and the process of grieving can be made up of our greatest cinematic moments. We all love cinema. Right? And therapeutically, whether working with the traumatic grief of a child who has lost a parent, or working with an adult client who has lost a spouse, or devastated by a sudden death, there are innate personal and emotional cinematic moments that can impact loss and mean the most. A child's impressionable drawings or watercolors or an adult's faraway look in the mind's eye of moments with a loved one is one's most innate ability to form pictures, evoke sound and words, or to remember a touch or gesture of the one lost. And the healing modality of cinema therapy based on the artistic rendering of film can (like no other art form) powerfully assist the process of grief. The great filmmaker Ingmar Berman said of the medium: "No form of art goes beyond ordinary consciousness as film does, straight to our emotions, deep into the twilight room of the soul" (Wolz, 2021, p.3). After many seasons of working with clients and grief from the approach of a companion, cinema therapy as adjunct or as a primary way of working with clients can shepherd individuals through the winter of grief.

What is the winter of grief? From my experience, it's when one's body of memories by the experience of the death of a loved one is still thawing, and when some parts of ourselves and our identity related to the beloved is still solid, not yet known to our fullest consciousness. This is when cinematic scenes selected for therapeutic impact can offer relief and perspective.

Characters, dialogue, settings and dramatic elements can assist with the unthawing, while at the same time offer a window of perspective and reflection that help individuals come to terms with loss as a reality and as a universal human experience. Through the use of films/movies, grief through imagery can be processed on the symbolic level that communicates from the subconscious to the conscious level activated by images (Wolz, 2021).

As a healing practitioner, this way of healing has been applied to my own grief experience. During the spring of 2020 after the sudden death of my 81-year-old mother, my identification of a scene in the film *Beasts of the Southern Wild* (2012) seen in the winter of the following year was powerfully cathartic. The scene depicted a young girl's bedside experience of the death of her earthy and fearless father while feeding him their favorite food. The heroic, beautiful and deeply painful scene between child and parent assisted to unearth my adult subconscious experience of my own mother's earthly and practical way of being my fearless parent, even in the moments near death. Additionally, a cinematic live theatrical scene that same season un-

What is the winter of grief? From my experience, it's when one's body of memories by the experience of the death of a loved one is still thawing, and when some parts of ourselves and our identity related to the beloved is still solid, not yet known to our fullest consciousness. This is when cinematic scenes selected for therapeutic impact can offer relief and perspective.

expectedly helped to crack open my pod of grief as well. Estranged in my grief, the thawing continued as the timeless Christmas character and psychic transformation of Ebenezer Scrooge in *A Christmas Carol* (The Old Vic, 2020) revealed my own transformation through the process of grief.

As ubiquitous as movie/film as product is since its commercial beginnings in the early part of the last century, as a tool of psychological and emotional healing, it is often categorized as sheer entertainment, particularly in American culture. The post-modern mega commercial success of the American film industry has too often regulated it as primarily a formulaic profit-making phenomenon, often dismissing and/or obscuring its value as a humanitarian art form that assists human evolution. Yet the mythical structure of narrative as a movie's primary agency is where the powerful therapeutic value lies. "Many cultures throughout human history have recognized the transforming and healing effect of the act of telling and listening to stories" (Wolz, 2021). Often after the loss of a loved one, one seeks one's own narrative in relation to the loss. Grief seeks out vignettes, stories within stories and indelible moments and themes of identification with the beloved. Selective cinema therapy can be the most important ingredient that starts the emotional thaw as the healing intervention that supports the most difficult moments in the winter of one's grief.

The Mythic Structure of Cinema and Working with Grief

I love cinema, and in my work with individuals and the grieving process, even when unrecognizable, human symbols are at play. As most humans on the planet have experienced a film/movie, in film the symbol as character, gesture, emotion or object can activate layers of experience that transport the experience of the individual to the universal and/or transpersonal, which can reflect the whole of humanity and common struggle and experience. This can be one of the important benefits of cinema therapy. Carl Jung said, "As the mind explores the symbol, it is led to ideas that lie beyond the grasp of reason" (Wolz, 2021). This state of unreason is often the experience of one who is grieving in which no amount of reason eases the pain of loss.

In work with a child, adolescent or adult in which cinema therapy is recommended, three conditions are needed to effectively apply the modality:

- assessing a client who is in the earliest season of grief in which emotions are raw and deeply hidden or denied, or in a later season of grief
- facilitating psycho-education that provides the client or client caregiver with the *why* of cinema therapy and how it works
- as facilitator, possessing a working understanding of the elements of cinema therapy and carefully selecting film titles/scenes that have been accessed to benefit the client's grieving process.

The primary elements of the film's narrative, character/s and actions should interpretively align with a client's own situation or emotional grieving process. Does a character express, encounter and/or struggle with death and/or loss in the film's narrative? What views and/or questions does the film raise in relation to death or the death of a loved one? Is the narrative related to an individual experience or a transpersonal one related to death? Is a film's theme or subtheme of death actual or metaphorical? Will the client be better served by viewing a film in which death is metaphorical versus actual? For example, in the epic film *The Lord of the Rings* (2001), the metaphorical death of the earth as it's known is a kind of cathartic rite of passage for the main characters of the narrative. This film example could perhaps best aid a client whose grief isn't acute, yet who is struggling with the spiritual meaning of death. Another example follows from the film *All Is Lost* (2013) in which the actual physical death of one man *almost* occurs, yet a spiritual death occurs in which he is redeemed and transformed. In these instances, the mystic structure of narrative supports a universal theme of death that can aid clients in the grief process suffering existential questions about the meaning of death after the actual loss of a loved one.

Selecting Films/Scenes for Cinema Therapy and Why

A key feature of working clinically with an application of cinema therapy is selecting films/movies that specifically hold the potential to aid grief. This also includes providing the client with an outline of how to view a selected film and allowing the client his/her experience of the film without the interference of the therapist's interpretation of the film. As important as a client's actual cathartic experience of a film while viewing may be, discussion with the therapist after viewing can also be critically and equally rich for supporting the client's grief process and powerful cathartic emotions. Introducing a client to a film, with psycho-education about films/movies as the healing modality, client film viewing and post-viewing discussion are all critical phases of the effectiveness of cinema therapy. Also unlike grief counseling in which the primary goal "is to help the survivor adapt to the loss of a loved one and...to adjust to a new reality with him or her" (Worden, 2009, p.84), grief therapy faces a different challenge. The goal of therapy is to help the mourner make "a better adaption to the loss" (Worden, 2009, p.153). It is through the process of cinema therapy that the better adaption is possible.

Preparing to work with a client by reviewing the basic principle of cinema therapy—that the mythic structure of film holds the potential of transformation and growth—is essential. A therapist's recall of his/her film viewing history and/or recommendation of a film from a colleague is a good start for cinematic film therapy selections. And it's required that therapists see all films/movies they recommend for supporting therapeutic safety for clients. Some films/movies (especially working with children and/or adolescents) can be inappropriate and even harmful to helping a client process his/her grief.

How to View a Selected Film for Processing Grief

The first question to ask related to your client is: What is the intensity of grief experienced by the client? Is the grief of loss still fresh, or is the client accepting of the loss and still considering its meaning? Is the client receptive to the modality of cinema healing, or would another approach work more effectively? Over what period of time would it be best to work with the client for navigating the natural process of grief through film? Ideally, if a client likes cinema, is informed by the nature of film as you provide psycho-education, and is willing to commit to the time to watch a film at least three times, the client can gain much from the intervention.

Here's an outline of the cathartic way (Wolz, 2021, p.22) of cinema therapy intervention:

1. Provide a session of psycho-education about cinema therapy. Explain the *why* of cinema therapy and client goals related.
2. Have the client select from a specific list of films prepared by the therapist, or perhaps the client has a film in mind.
3. Instruct the client to do a first viewing alone without thinking about any element of the film, but just for relaxation and/or enjoyment.
4. Afterwards, instruct the client to watch the film again for a character she/he most identifies with and to consider why. Is it a direct scene of death/loss or the circumstances that led to it that are most impactful for the client? How does a main character respond to or cope with death?
5. Facilitate a post-viewing discussion with the client about the film— characters, scenes and settings—and how these relate to his/her grief experience. Encourage the client to name their own experience of the film.

Primarily, the role of the therapist is to assist the client in bringing alive their most impactful and cathartic experiences of film characters and/or scenes with interpreting. Help the client to clarify reactions, identification with a specific character and recognition with no need to be a film critic and/or expert. Remind the client of his/her opportunity to make sense of death and loss through the experience of the film. As therapist, mirror the client's experience with empathic presence.

Cinema Therapy Grief Healing with Expressive Body Writing

As an expressive arts practitioner and licensed psychotherapist, I find adding interventions such as making art in conjunction with cinema therapy further extends the potential impact on a client's grief. Cinema therapy is an expressive modality in which each client suffering the experience of grief will have a unique experience of his/her engagement with film and interpretation of it based on their experience of loss.

Additionally, as a practitioner, I have developed a therapeutic expressive writing intervention that clients are invited to after a selected film is decided upon with which to work with the client's grief, as mentioned earlier. The process from the perspective of practitioner is one of a companion to the client versus an expert or teacher. My decided personal approach was developed after working with children and their families for many months in a hospital program to aid children who had lost parents by sudden illness, suicide, homicide or accident. The work with this population and their families provided me with an understanding of grief as a natural process and one innately specific to humans of all ages. I observed that minimal, empathic, non-intrusive, yet professionally informed facilitation of the grief process best served those suffering the loss of a loved one. During that time I walked alongside my clients in their grief on the paths they knew best. As leading grief educator, author and developer of the companioning grief model Alan Wolfelt (2022) states of the role of therapist and/or counselor, "Their role is not to try and fix it, or to give you un-asked for advice. Their role is to be there, actively listen and to offer their love and presence."

Grief Writing Intervention

As a child and family therapist and professional creative writer, I have experienced for decades the firsthand benefits of expressive writing and its power to heal. Working with writing onto paper as an expressive medium allows for a greater space of the client experience and psychological exploration of grief by use of spontaneity and gentle guidance. Writing is also a somatic practice, in that writing through the body itself offers transforming benefits. As expressive writing innovator and researcher James Pennebaker (2020) reveals about his ground-breaking expressive writing study in 1986, benefits experienced by study participants included "decreased anxiety, blood pressure, depression, muscle tension, pain and stress." These benefits I have also witnessed working with clients as an added feature of cinema therapy for grief.

Once you get the client's agreement and receptivity to writing in therapy, ask that they purchase a journal for writing and bring it to the session after watching a selected film. Once in session, ask the client about their initial impression of the film. Was it like other films viewed recently or not so recently? Was the film easy to follow? Did it capture their attention from the start? Then ask the client to watch the film again, especially watching characters that they most identify with. While watching, instruct the client to write in response to a character, and what a character does, and dialogue (or scenes of dialogue) that speak to the client's experience of grief.

Inform the client that there's no right or wrong way to do it, except to capture honest language that speaks to their cathartic experience of grief through viewing the film.

Instruct the client to watch the film a third time in which they write for sensory experience, content and insight. Invite them to *feel* their experience of the film through their own words written on paper.

Have a final post session in which the client shares his/her experience of the film and *their writing* to explore deeper reactions to the film and his/her cathartic experience of his/her own grief.

Film Recommendations for Working with Grief and Catharsis

There are many, many films that can be suitable for working with a client and/or family with the issue of grief. When a practitioner recommends a film/movie viewing to a client, it should be recommended as a whole viewing experience in addition to therapeutic exploration. As a post-therapeutic exercise, it can be suggested to clients that they create a list of their own films in addition to films selected in therapy for future reference.

Recent and not-so-recent films (most recent first):

Death/Dying/Loss
- Mucchino, G. (Director) (2015). *Fathers and Daughters* [Film]. Vertical Entertainment.
- Posin, A. (Director) (2014). *The Face of Love* [Film]. IFC Films.
- Boone, J. (Director) (2014). *The Fault in Our Stars* [Film]. 20th Century Studios.
- McQueen, S. (Director) (2013). *12 Years a Slave* [Film]. Searchlight Pictures.
- Chandor, J.C. (Director) (2013). *All Is Lost* [Film]. Lionsgate Films.
- Zeitlin, B. (Director) (2012). *Beasts of the Southern Wild* [Film]. Searchlight Pictures.
- Parker, O. (Director) (2012). *Now Is Good* [Film]. Warner Bros. Pictures.

- Blume, L. (Director) (2012). *Tiger Eyes* [Film]. Sonoma International Film Festival.
- Crowe, C. (Director) (2011) *We Bought a Zoo* [Film]. 20th Century Studios.
- Payne, A. (Director) (2011). *The Descendants* [Film]. Searchlight Pictures.
- LaBute, N. (Director) (2010). *Death at a Funeral* [Film]. Screen Gems.
- Eastwood, C. (Director) (2010). *Hereafter* [Film]. Warner Bros. Pictures.
- Cassavetes, N. (Director) (2009). *My Sister's Keeper* [Film]. Warner Bros. Pictures.
- Doctor, P. (Director) (2009). *Up* [Film]. Walt Disney Pictures.
- Csupó, G. (Director) (2007). *A Bridge to Terabithia* [Film]. Walden Media.
- Reiner, R. (Director) (2007). *The Bucket List* [Film]. Warner Bros. Pictures.
- Bier, S. (Director) (2007). *Things We Lost in the Fire* [Film]. Paramount Pictures.
- Lee, A. (Director) (2005) *Brokeback Mountain* [Film]. Paramount Pictures.
- Forster, M. (Director) (2004). *Finding Neverland.* [Film]. Miramax.
- Zhang, Y. (Director) (2004). *House of Flying Daggers* [Film]. Warner Bros. Pictures.
- Amenábar, A. (Director) (2004). *The Sea Inside* [Film]. Warner Bros. Pictures.
- Shankman, A. (Director) (2002). *A Walk to Remember* [Film]. Warner Bros. Pictures.
- Jackson, P. (Director) (2001). *The Lord of the Rings* [Film]. New Line Cinema.
- Eyre, C. (Director) (1998). *Smoke Signals* [Film]. Miramax.
- Singelton, J. (Director) (1991). *Boyz n the Hood* [Film]. Columbia Pictures.
- Dash, J. (Director) (1991). *Daughters of the Dust* [Film]. Kino International.
- Zucker, J. (Director) (1990). *Ghost* [Film]. Paramount Pictures.
- Weir, P. (Director) (1989). *Dead Poet's Society* [Film]. Touchstone Pictures.
- Ross, H. (Director) (1989). *Steel Magnolias* [Film]. Sony Pictures.

- Imamura, S. (Director) (1983). *The Ballad of Narayama* [Film]. Toei Company.
- Rydell, M. (Director) (1981). *On Golden Pond* [Film]. Metro-Goldwyn-Mayer.
- Kulik, B. (Director) (1971). *Brian's Song* [Film]. American Broadcasting Company.
- Hiller, A. (Director) (1970). *Love Story* [Film]. Paramount Pictures.
- Berman, I. (Director). (1958). *The Seventh Seal* [Film]. AB Svensk Filmindustri.
- Stevenson, R. (Director) (1957). *Old Yeller* [Film]. Walt Disney Pictures.

Films Suitable for Children

(Many of the above films listed are also suitable for adolescents and children with adult supervision.)

- Unkrich, L. (Director) (2017). *Coco* [Film]. Walt Disney Studios.
- Moore, T. (Director) (2014). *Song of the Sea* [Film]. Studio Canal.

References

Chandor, J.C. (2013). *All Is Lost* [Film]. Lionsgate/Roadside Attractions.

Jackson, P. (2001–2003). *The Lord of the Rings* [Film Series]. New Line Cinema/WingNut Films.

Pennebaker, J. (2020). Write your secrets: What James Pennebaker discovered about expressive writing. The Change Companies. www.changecompanies.net/blog/james-pennebaker-expressive-writing

The Old Vic. (2020). *A Christmas Carol* [Live Theatrical Performance]. Old Vic Theatre, London.

Wolfelt, A. (2022) Getting help. Center for Loss and Life Transition. www.centerforloss.com/grief/getting-help

Wolz, B. (2021). *Cinema Therapy: Using the Power of Imagery in Films for the Therapeutic Process.* California: Zur Institute.

Worden, W.J. (2009). *Counselling and Grief Therapy: A Handbook for the Mental Health Practitioner.* New York, NY: Routledge.

Zeitlin, B. (2012). *Beasts of the Southern Wild* [Film]. Fox Searchlight.

CHAPTER 9

Drawing Deeper Realms

The Touch Drawing Process

Deborah Koff-Chapin

Touch Drawing is a simple yet profound way of creating images through the touch of fingertips on paper. It has been my core creative practice since I came upon it in revelatory play in 1974.

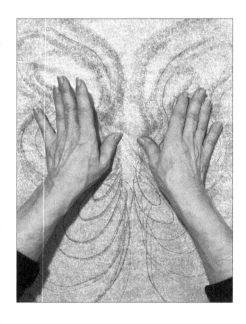

I begin by rolling out paint on a board and placing paper upon it. Gazing at the blank sheet of paper, I turn my focus inward. I feel as blank as the paper. I wait, scanning my body for a rising impulse. I feel a longing in my heart. It begins to take shape. My hands touch the paper and move in alignment with this felt sense, creating marks on the underside of the page through the pressure of my touch. I come to stillness again, feeling into what may grow from this initial gesture. I become aware of my shoulders and trace a sense of them around the first gesture. I continue feeling for the image from the inside out. Gradually an expressive figure emerges from the initial gesture. Lifting the paper off the board, I see the marks created by the pressure of my touch on the paint below. I glance at the drawing and lay it aside. Picking up my roller, I smooth out the paint, erasing any record of the previous drawing in the paint. I lift a new sheet of paper and let it float down onto the board. I gaze at the blank sheet, turn inward and scan my sensations once again. Over and over, I continue this rhythm, as images emerge from within onto the page. It is an inner journey. When I come to a sense of completion, I look through the series of drawings that have just emerged, witnessing the transformation I have just taken myself through.

Touch Drawing has been there for me in the most challenging and the most inspiring seasons of my life. In the early days, my psyche was vulnerable and unstable. I would sit at my drawing board and scratch raw feelings onto paper, continuing until I found a sense of presence and stability. Last week after hiking up a dramatic trail on Mount Baker, I sat in awe. Although it felt impossible to encompass, I stretched myself open, translating something of its glacial presence through my body and onto paper.

And then there are the thresholds of life and death. I brought my Touch Drawing materials to the hospital for the birth of my daughter in 1986. It was a long labor. In the middle of the night, I sat at the drawing board. As each contraction came over me like a wave, I let it pass through my body, out of my fingertips and onto the paper. As I embraced the experience with a sense of creation, my relationship to the pain of the contractions shifted. Their intensity was diluted as they expanded throughout and beyond my body. These

The expressive arts give us a safe space where we can become more comfortable with opening to the unknown. This enables us to more fully trust the process of life, through its joys and sorrows. Creative expression taps deeper realms of wisdom and possibility.

were the easiest contractions of my 32-hour labor. And I now have a visual record of this life passage—direct impressions of my labor and of my daughter being born.

I have only given birth once. But I have done Touch Drawing around the deaths of quite a few people. When I hear of a loved one who is near the threshold or recently passed, I often feel called to be present through Touch Drawing. The impulse to draw comes as a quiet urging—a subtle feeling of connection. It is a way to make space for deeper attention. It can be a time of creative prayer and a way to offer support to loved ones. Sometimes I give the drawings to family. Other times I keep these "threshold drawings" private—sensing that they are better left as an engagement between myself and the soul who has passed.

As I was preparing to write about Touch Drawing at the threshold of life and death, a synchronistic connection occurred. I notice a new post on the Facebook Touch Drawing group. It was by Susan Arnsten-Russell, a long-time practitioner and facilitator of Touch Drawing. She posted a series of drawings that she had just created along with these words.

> Someone I know, someone whose life has intertwined with mine for more than 40 years, is dying. Touch Drawing provides the tools to process what this means to me and to draw in service for this family member.

Someone commented on the post, saying how true they found this to be and shared that Touch Drawing had helped them in a recent bereavement, and had eased the pain of their loved one's passing.

It was touching for me to witness this affirming interaction, especially as I was amid writing about just this. I called Susan and we talked about the experience of doing Touch Drawing in attunement to deeper layers of life. She articulated something that I also experience. "It doesn't feel like I am really connecting in the moment. I just trust the process and do it. But when I look back at the drawings and the words I wrote, I realize they really do get to the heart of the matter."

Trusting the process—this is what I continue to practice as I do Touch Drawing. The expressive arts give us a safe space where we can become more comfortable with opening to the unknown. This enables us to more fully trust the process of life, through its joys and sorrows. Creative expression taps deeper realms of wisdom and possibility. They are a birthright of human life. Find your art form and trust the process.

Find out more about Touch Drawing at https://touchdrawing.com.

CHAPTER 10

Walking Therapy

Exploring Our Inner World Through Our Outer World
Louise Allen

Introduction

I would like to clarify that you do not need to walk to engage in this process. It is important to recognise that there are barriers to walking therapy for many people, and not everyone who may benefit from this process walks as their way of travelling in the world. As someone who walks as my way of engaging in this process, this is the perspective from which I have reflected. However, I also sometimes climb, sit, crawl, fidget, run, stomp and drive. Sometimes I am a passenger, sometimes I am driving. There is rich discussion among outdoor therapists around the terminology for "walking therapy," with some preferring to use the term "outdoor or eco therapy" to better include people who do not walk.

Some therapists opt for the term "walk and talk," valuing the accessibility of the clarity of the term, while others find it reductive and dismissive of the active role of the natural environment. "Walking therapy" felt like the best, if not ideal, fit for this section as this intervention explores the journeying aspect of the therapeutic process: from one to another, the space between, the pace and gait. For this reason, I wanted to use a word that captured the idea of travelling, of moving through.

In other-than-human nature in winter, I see the final flurries of the busyness of autumn—last-minute frantic gatherings of squirrels, leaves whipped by the wind, finally frozen and forced from their branches. A quieter, emptier, slower time. Darker, colder, more exposing conditions. Animals hibernating or conserving energy. Going inward: into burrows, nests, building up fat reserves to create a buffer from the cold and sparseness.

One of the defining qualities of winter is the shorter hours of daylight and longer darkness.

Even during daylight hours, shadows are longer in the winter as the wintering area of the earth is tilted away from the sun. In *Becoming Animal* (2010), David Abram explores how we are used to thinking of our shadow as a two dimensional "kinetic pancake" of flatness. In actuality, "shadow is an enigma more substantial than that flat shape on the paved ground...it is a voluminous being of thickness and depth, a mostly unseen presence that dwells in the air between my body and that ground."

Just as darkness is present in the world around us, it is also within us—a part of life, of our being. When we think of our inner darkness, we may think of it in many different ways. Perhaps the parts of ourselves that are not yet known to ourselves, that we have not seen? Or maybe the parts of us we hide and do not want others to see. Perhaps we think of our inner darkness as uncomfortable feelings or situations we perceive as intolerable that try to shut out of our awareness. Or an emptiness in the absence or void of what we had, or what we want. Whatever it means to you, if we approach the idea of our emotional or psychological darkness in grief with a perspective of depth, we have a whole dimension to explore.

I have come to think that some of the gifts of winter are, in fact, the bleakness, the darkness and the stillness. The time of emptiness and where life slows right down. It can be a dark and challenging time to tolerate in an emotional sense—the really feeling the starkness of what is no longer there, of the loss. And when our external world is in winter, and is quieter and darker, we might be less distracted away from the weight of our personal experience. And yet, where other animals and plants conserve energy in the winter to enable them to re-emerge in spring, perhaps an inner winter gives us an opportunity to become more acquainted with that sadness and darkness and hold ourselves through it. It is sometimes said that the size of our sadness, our anger, our envy is somehow in tune with what we love, what we believe in, what we long for. When we listen to our pain, it often holds a message about what is really important to us and what we need. When we know this, we can begin to find ways to both recognise and honour what we love(d) and begin to prepare for how we can meet our needs as we emerge from our own winter.

I used to think of myself as a fair-weather outdoor lover until I tried walking outside in the wind and the rain and on the overcast days, and I realised I could love the outdoors then, too. For me, this resonated as a metaphor for welcoming in and being with less comfortable emotions—grief, anger, jealousy and fear. There was something quite transformative about connecting my outer bodily experience in the physical world with my inner bodily experience and emotional world. I realised that there was a subtle connection with how I related to being outdoors when it was wet, windy and cold, and how I related to feeling certain emotions. In essence, if it's not comfortable or I can't see the obvious beauty or reason for it, avoid it or find somewhere more comfortable and wait until the sun comes out. Physically, this meant I was generally warmer, drier and had a loving and enthusiastic relationship with nature and the outdoors.

Psychologically, I felt depths of joy, excitement, gratitude, relaxation and optimism and was generally comfortable. And, as the connection came into focus whilst walking unprepared in the mud with ill-fitting shoes and heavy rain with no waterproof coat, I realised I had been missing the exhilaration of finding shelter from the downpour, the frustration, temporary fear and sense of achievement of being stuck in the mud and finding a way through. I realised that if I never felt into the less comfortable emotional feelings, I would be missing the complexity of what they held. Jumping straight into those uncomfortable and seemingly terrifying feelings wasn't possible—my psyche seemed well practised at diverting me away from this forbidden well of feeling. So I decided that if I couldn't easily journey into these parts of my inner landscape, I would practise walking in a less comfortable outer landscape.

It did take some reluctant embracing of waterproof trousers and some experimenting with walking boots along the way. It doesn't always feel "good," and on the longer, wet walks or the times the rain or wind catches me un-awares, there is often sweary muttering to myself and gritted teeth. Yet I now know I can find beauty, meaning and even sometimes joy when I embrace those times. It feels liberating to be able to journey and know I can survive it; that the relentless downpour, or the ankle-deep wading through mud, or the aching muscles or the vastness between me and where I want to be will change.

Gradually, I found this approach to navigating the physical world (along with the patience and empathy of friends and the skill of some great thera-pists) helped me to find ways to accompany myself in a way of being in my inner world. It's an ongoing practice of patience with myself, courage and getting to know where, when and who I need to be around to journey into those parts of myself, or to stay there when I find myself there unexpectedly.

Just as darkness is present in the world around us, it is also within us—a part of life, of our being.

We can shut out and avoid the cold, the darkness, the discomfort or inconvenience of nature's unpredictability. Indeed, in our Western culture we often tend to do just that—with electric lighting, and central heating, and working patterns that resist the waning light and warmth calling us to stop and slow down, we can pretend that the discomfort and limitations of the winter are not happening. This can be protective and comforting, it can circumnavigate or ease frustrations, it might mean we are productive and get things done, and it can mean we miss the opportunity to really experience the fullness of winter and what it is to live through the cold with conscious awareness. Katherine May discusses the idea of "Wintering" in her book of the same name (2020)—exploring how we might understand and embrace our environmental and inner winters, and what gifts and learning are to be found when we do.

We often relate to physical winter in the UK in parallel with the way we relate to grief—the darker, colder, more raw feelings. We generally don't approach grief with arms and heart open, with sadness for others to witness, support and share in. We feel the need to protect ourselves and others from the depth of our pain, constraining the emotion as we do it. In *The Wild Edge of Sorrow* (2015), Francis Weller identifies this privacy of pain as a commonly Western way of grieving, not shared across all cultures where ritual and communal processing of grief is more commonplace. Approaching the well of grief as a rich opportunity to learn what gifts it holds for us is a position taken by many therapists; we strive to create a space safe enough for someone to begin to lean into and allow the depth of their emotion. A space that is often not reflected in wider society, though attitudes are slowly changing.

If we think of those raw moments of grief as a deep ocean, a dark thicket or a cold winter. Think of the depths of sadness and loss, of anguish and sorrow as the harshness and sparseness of a cold, harsh and dark winter climate. It takes resilience, preparation and bracing to weather the winter. Continuing the emotional metaphor, I see a connection here with relearning how to feel our feelings, tuning in to how we are really doing. And with nurturing safe and trusting relationships—whether that be with oneself, with friends, with family, a bereavement support group or with a therapist. When the winter of grief comes around, for however long it may last, we are able to be with its wildness and hear and learn from the depth of our loss, and have the reserves and resources within ourselves and support around us to help us through.

When we want to explore or understand the frostiness within us—emerging from our hibernation, if you like—the safety of the therapeutic relationship and space can enable us to do so. Perhaps it also takes hope and a desire to find a reason to come through the other side into spring. Walking therapy offers an opportunity to move, at the person's own physical pace and gait, while exploring their inner world, including any stuckness or stillness, thereby inviting in some movement, like a physical thawing, which often enables more of a flow of thoughts, feelings and emotions. The following method uses an exploration of physical movement, of pace and gait, as a catalyst to understand and reflect on our emotional and psychological experience.

Planning a Walking Therapy Session

Know Your Area

Working outdoors, particularly when walking or moving through a space, extends the physical boundary of the therapeutic space horizontally. It also extends the physical boundary vertically, introducing unpredictability in the weather and the terrain—dry paths may be firm underfoot in the summer but quickly become muddy in the rain. I recommend getting to know the outdoor space or route you will use prior to working therapeutically outdoors. This will help you to hold the space safely and enable you to anticipate some of the potential challenges, opportunities and changes of the space.

Physical Suitability

It is important to consider and assess how the person's physical ability aligns with the physical terrain and environment. Anticipating and planning for a walking therapy session can be a rich opportunity in itself for collaborative exploration when thinking about the suitability of a location to walk. It may raise issues around mobility, access and inclusion, for example. Consider access to toilets, public transport, parking and other facilities, allergies and how the person feels about dogs, horses or other animals you may encounter.

Psychological Suitability

As well as the terrain, before working outdoors, consider the person's existing relationship to certain environments and outdoor spaces. Are they aware of any past experiences which may come up outdoors? How do they feel about privacy and the potential for briefly being overheard by passers-by? Do they have any phobias or concerns that may affect working outdoors?

A Fellow Traveller

You literally become a fellow traveller as a therapist in walking therapy (not purely metaphorically as per Irvin Yalom's definition (2017)). How you take up this literal role is just as relevant as it is psychologically when working relationally with someone in therapy.

How will you decide where you walk, and why? Consider whether you will determine and lead the route, or hold the time boundary alone and let the route be determined by the person having counselling. How much will you bring in your own observations and knowledge of the natural space and the person? Might you invite or suggest someone changes the way they move either to suit you or their interests?

Taking a Witness Approach

Taking a witness approach led by the person having counselling, notice how they are moving while they talk and invite them to reflect on the way they are moving. Questions or observations may include:

- I notice you seem flustered. How has your journey here been? How does it feel to arrive here? (e.g. at the beginning of a session)
- What do you notice about the speed we've been walking at? Does that say anything about what we have been talking about? (e.g. on noticing that you are out of breath or finding the pace more comfortable yourself)
- We are about halfway through the session. How is it to be here? (this could be interpreted and explored in many ways, here in the physical place, here in the content of the session, here in the duration of the session, here in the position in a regular route)
- What was it like for you to have got round that puddle/dodged that wave/been diverted by the fallen tree/been soaked in the rain last week, etc.? (e.g. if you have navigated an unexpected or challenging area)
- How does it feel to decide which way we will walk? (e.g. if they are leading the direction of the route)

- Thinking about how you were walking during the session, is there anything you notice? Does that relate to what you were talking about throughout the session? (e.g. at the end of a session or when bringing a session to a close—perhaps they started the session walking very fast, feeling anxious or stressed, and their pace slowed throughout as they feel calmer)
- We seem to have arrived back earlier/later than usual. How has this session been for you? (e.g. at the end of a session when walking a regular route)

Some Movement- and Walking-Related Descriptive Words

Wandering	Dragging	Rolling
Meandering	Dancing	Stomping
Striding	Floating	Steering
Exploring	Daydreaming	Tumbling
Trudging	Determining	Falling
Tiptoeing	Crawling	Leading
Creeping	Bounding	Following

Taking a Facilitative Approach

You may also invite the person to explore what comes up for them, what happens to their emotional and psychological world when they change the way they move their physical body. This might look like:

If the person has racing thoughts, is overwhelmed by "things to do" or talks through how they are very fast, with little time and space to allow feelings to emerge, you might invite them to intentionally slow their pace and breathing. Invite them to reflect: How does it feel physically/emotionally/mentally to slow your walking pace?

If you notice they have said something significant, you have noticed incongruence or you intuit that they are brushing past something important, you might invite them to pause and stop walking completely for a moment. Invite them to share how it feels to pause. What comes up in the space the stillness creates?

Choose your timing and location mindfully when slowing and pausing as this can open up space for otherwise suppressed and avoided emotions to surface.

If someone is feeling depressed, depleted or struggling with motivation, you might invite them to intentionally pick up the pace. You could do this verbally or invite an increased pace by walking faster yourself and noticing whether they pick up their pace to match yours. After walking for a while, invite reflection such as "How is our walking pace feeling?" Invite the person to consider whether the pace has any effect on how they feel emotionally.

You might collaboratively identify a need or desire for playfulness or lightness.

Depending on your location, you could ask, "How would it feel to stomp through those muddy puddles?" "You mention how enticing the sea looks—I wonder how it would be to take y/our shoes off and paddle?" "That tree looks pretty good for climbing..."

The invitation or suggestion might not be taken up immediately, but by bringing the option in, you are showing that you welcome those parts of the person, too.

You might combine both witness and facilitative approaches collaboratively with the person, asking what they'd prefer or need from you to find the session most helpful.

How and When It Can Be Used

Walking therapy can be experienced as less intense than sitting in a room facing one another as, generally, you are side by side or in front of one another. This can enable some people to speak more freely than they might indoors. Additionally, for those who find it easier to talk while they are fiddling with something or colouring, the physical process of walking and distraction in other nature can enable some people to focus more easily on communicating thoughts and feelings.

As with all approaches, the environment, the smells, sounds, noises and potential for passing others will be enabling for some; for others, working outdoors might be overwhelming and inhibiting.

Working outdoors in the vaster space can also feel too open and too unpredictable for some people. A more closely contained space, either indoors or finding a sheltered area to sit outdoors, might be more conducive to opening up. Be led by the individual and check in regularly to review how helpful the way of working is.

Although the introduction to this way of working refers to the potential benefits of walking as a way of easing the psychological movement of "stuck" or uncomfortable emotions, this technique can be used at any time to give the opportunity to reflect on how physical movement and navigation through the external world may enable awareness of inner processes.

To deepen an understanding of how it feels to be in a psychological or emotional winter, you might initially take more of a witness approach (as above), tuning in to where someone is currently at, what it is like to be there. If you have an existing depth to your therapeutic relationship, or a depth of self-awareness, a more facilitative approach may follow and encourage further depth, moving beyond conscious awareness and exploring what might be underneath coping strategies.

Different therapists may choose to approach walking therapy from two different positions, or interchange between the two:

- **A human-centric perspective** of positioning humans as more important than other-than-human life and viewing nature as a space to be utilised. This might include taking a more traditional indoor therapeutic approach outside.
- **An eco-centric perspective**, positioning humans, other-than-human beings and the landscape, weather and other aspects of nature as all equally valuable and important in the therapeutic process.

My personal philosophy is positioned in a more eco-centric approach to life, and this underpins and informs the exercise above. However, the extent to which I bring in observations and invitations to connect and explore relationship with the natural world when I am counselling varies, depending on the individual hopes, preferences, values and focus of the person I am working with.

Walking therapy is also just one option in the broad field of outdoor therapy which includes wilderness therapy, gardening/horticultural therapy, animal-assisted therapy and more. The exploration above is just one opportunity that working outdoors brings—there are an increasing number of outdoor and walking therapy training courses, workshops and qualifications offered to explore the field further.

References

Abram, D. (2010). *Becoming Animal: An Earthly Cosmology*. New York, NY: Vintage Books.

May, K. (2020). *Wintering: The Power of Rest and Retreat in Difficult Times*. London: Ebury Publishing.

Weller, F. (2015). *The Wild Edge of Sorrow: Rituals of Renewal and the Sacred Work of Grief*. Huichin, unceded Ohlone land, aka Berkeley, CA: North Atlantic Books.

Yalom, I. (2017). *The Gift of Therapy: An Open Letter to a New Generation of Therapists and Their Patients*. New York, NY: Harper.

PART THREE

SPRING

Awakening

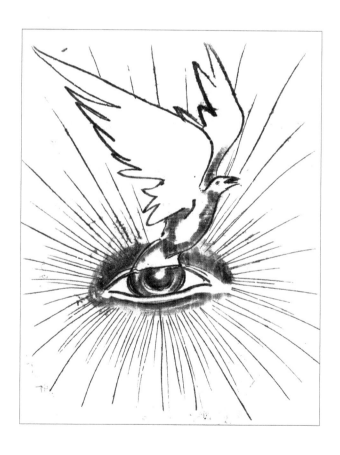

Coming Through

Fall silent and you will hear it growing,
insistent as grass through asphalt.
You know it has always been there,
pregnant with possibility, finding
form. Now it is coming through,
seeking light,
earning a visible place
in this world you have made.

Listen.
Like a known voice in a crowded
room it will come,
follow the silver thread
of attention to reach your
ear. It only requires
attunement,
a paring away of
excess to hear the
pure tone.

Like sculpting hands
you must work the
substance to find its
essential form.
There is something inside the
mass for which your life is the
template, awaiting the accident
of discovery. Now you must caress
its naked shape, shiver at its
frailty,
know its strength.

All you have been has readied
you for this becoming.

~ Robert A. Neimeyer

Spring Reflection

Claudia Coenen

In spring, the plants burst up through the moist soil and birds and small animals appear. The air is fresh again, and we can gather together, wandering down a woodland path or meeting at a sidewalk café. "Hello," we say. "It's so nice to see you! How have you been?" We sit down together, under a tree or in brightly colored folding chairs, and invite a story.

We are storied beings. We narrate our lives to each other and even to ourselves as we move through each day. We shape our lives in anecdotes, explanations, memories of past events and interactions. When someone dies, we say to each other "Remember that time when he..." or "This was her favorite dish; I remember how she closed her eyes in delight the first time she tasted it."

Spring is a wistful time for me because it is Alby time. His birthday was May 6th and he died on May 10th, four days after his 50th birthday. In my garden and the gardens of all my sisters, there is a bleeding-heart plant, which always blooms in May. Our bleeding-hearts are cuttings from the one his sister planted in her garden right after he died. Lilacs send out their heady perfume in May as well, and Alby, a gardener at heart, loved lilacs and all the flowers of spring.

In the early years of grief, spring was a difficult time for all of us who loved Alby. Now, so many years later, I am gladdened by the reminders of his presence and love all the flowers that are connected to him. My bleeding-heart has grown from a single plant to a patch of many, arching its pink and white hearts over its palmate foliage.

My love for him continues even though he is gone. I miss him. Still.

The birds always wake me up before daybreak. Chirping, swooping and rustling in the leaves outside, they are foraging to fatten up before the season turns. They've spent the summer season building nests and raising new families. Now they will leave their temporary homes, fly elsewhere and start anew. Their activity is the cycle: build, nurture and release, repeating over and over.

I don't remember listening so intently to the early birds before my husband died. Afterwards, I would wonder, how could they sing so loudly, when he was no longer here? I looked out the window, surprised that he was not wandering outside in the dawn. Now, so many years later, I cannot listen to the sounds of the dawn without missing his lean frame, head tilted back to squint at the sky, cup of coffee in his hand.

CHAPTER 11

Caregiving and Grieving as Creative Process

A Conversation with Ilana Rowe

Dorit Netzer

The tulips in my garden
Do not fade all at once
They may lose a few petals
Before their sun-kissed heads
Wrinkle with a farewell to spring.
All life is passing.
And what we know to be ephemeral
Is cherished all the more.

~ Dorit Netzer

This chapter is the culmination of the author's collaboration with Ilana Rowe, through conversation and creative expression, exploring subtle dimensions in the lived experience of her creative and spiritual journey of grief. Ilana and I have been long-time colleagues and friends, with similar clinical practices as well as educational and teaching backgrounds in transpersonal psychology and the expressive arts. We have taken a co-creative, dialectic approach to sharing a glimpse into Ilana's journey of caregiving her husband Hal and grieving his loss to Alzheimer's disease, with the intention to deepen our understanding of her experience in a way that would ultimately inform others.

We began by contemplating how to structure an interview about Ilana's creative nonfiction memoir *Sacred Stories: A Caregiver's Journey Through Alzheimer's* (Rowe, 2020), and expanded upon it through shared reflections, to provide additional insight regarding the language of imagery and creative expression as vehicles for the grieving process. Our hope was that her journey will resonate with art therapists and other caregivers on a personal level, as a way to explore their own experiences of grief and loss and suggest a creative approach to accompanying the grieving process of others as a participatory witness.

Ilana's memoir (Rowe, 2020), which she wrote the year following her husband's death, reveals the nonlinear manner in which her creative expression and attunement to the mystical in living and dying have ushered her through grieving her loss of Hal and remembering their lives during a decade of encountering the progressive symptoms of Alzheimer's. With her anticipatory grief, which emerged during the mid to late stages of Hal's Alzheimer's, Ilana's heart-centered practices, creativity, and intuition made it possible to notice the sacred in both life and death.

Dialogue, Imagery, and Deep Listening

In a similar manner to prior creative collaborations I conducted with artists and transpersonal scholars (Netzer, 2016, 2017), the following dialogue was structured as the container for a collegial exchange, with the intention to generate a third dimension of shared awareness about creative exploration, imagery, synchronicity, and attunement with the natural world in the midst of grieving. These imaginal and mystical dimensions of her lived experience not only permeated Ilana's journey but also shaped the ways in which our collaboration unfolded.

We utilized a qualitative method of inquiry that acknowledges all involved as co-researchers—equal participants in the search and re-search for meaning. In this approach, a dialogic form of interviewing (Way, Zwier, & Tracy, 2015) is followed by a collaborative processing of the interview transcript (Creswell & Miller, 2000) and the disclosure of as much of the transcript as possible to the reader. By including our conversation verbatim in this chapter, we not only attempt to preserve the authenticity of our respective voices but also invite the reader to join us as a co-researcher and participatory witness (Netzer, 2017).

In the tradition of transpersonal inquiry (Anderson & Braud, 2011), all who participate in this process might emerge with insight, a sense of discovery, and personal transformation. We believe that this form of exploratory dialogue can be employed among colleagues, as well as have its applications when working with clients, to cultivate deep listening, reflexivity, and awareness of transference and countertransference in response to the existential and spiritual aspects of life and death. The return to a recorded conversation and a written transcript provides both speaker and listener the opportunity to witness self and other, uncover additional layers of thoughts and feelings, and honor the dynamic nature of grieving.

As I prepared for my conversation with Ilana, a few questions about the purpose of this joint exploration emerged. What will we gain and lose in this process? Will it connect us more deeply with life and with those we each lost? Will it prepare us further for our continued life journeys and for that which remains a mystery? What might emerge through our collaboration that could not have transpired without it? As I wrote these questions down, I recognized that I was not seeking immediate answers, but wished to hold all these questions with awe as we began this journey together. We looked forward to exploring creative expression as a container for healing and meaning making during the lived experience of Alzheimer's heartbreaking inevitability, or as Ilana put it, "breathe new life into the understanding of the process."

The Interview

As much as our process was set up as a collegial collaboration, our roles were unique. While the focus of the conversation is one person's experience, the interviewer brings up questions and follows up with interpretive comments that depend on and are restricted by prior personal and professional experiences (Netzer, 2016, 2017). The collaboration is therefore acknowledged from the outset as inter-subjective (Roulston, 2010). As in other forms of self-reflective dialogues, such as between the therapist and client, I have done my best to observe the inescapable tendency of projecting my own experience, in the process of attempting to be empathically present to Ilana's vulnerable recollections. With keen awareness of the pitfalls of transference, we recognized the impact of shared discoveries as a transformative opportunity to integrate new ways of seeing generated within this creative encounter (May, 1975/1994).

We would be remiss to not mention prior to presenting excerpts from the interview that our first conversation took place shortly after the news of Russia's invasion of Ukraine. Our compassion for the many lives lost abroad colored the tone of our dialogue and amplified how no personal loss is without reverberation in the collective. We began with a centering practice through self-observation, imagination, and drawing, in which we first grounded ourselves by paying attention to details in our physical environments that early March morning (Ilana in Florida and Dorit in New York), and then gave form to our respective inner landscapes through quick, expressive drawings. The rest of the conversation unfolded organically, following the thread of our shared intention to grow through this collaboration and remain open to the mystery of not knowing, the "spirit in-between…the creative source of our being" (Ferrer, 2011, pp.3–23). In this process of mutual attunement, as Ilana shared her story and described the images that guided her along the way, I paid attention to images, insight, and the felt sense that emerged within me in resonance with her journey.

Attunement and Imaginal Resonance

Dorit Netzer (DN): I want to begin this conversation by grounding ourselves and telling each other about our physical surroundings. What is it like this morning where you are?

Ilana Rowe (IR): It's pretty overcast in Florida today. It's beautiful weather. Probably 75 degrees. Where I live is so beautiful and lush and forested. I live right next to a most beautiful oak tree, the oldest one in our community; it's deeded never to be cut down. I wrote about this tree in my book. She was a teacher for me. Grandmother trees like this remind me that the aging process can be beautiful.

When I discovered that this particular place was available, I sold the unit where Hal and I lived together and bought this one. Changing my living space was really important for my grieving process. In my first place, there were so many reminders of living with Alzheimer's. The new one gave me a fresh start.

DN: Your description takes me back to my visit five years ago. Hal was already significantly impacted by Alzheimer's progression, but I remember the two of you and your puppy, Oliver, enjoying a moment of joy and laughter.

IR: Yes, and I was lucky, he always remained gentle and sweet even as his Alzheimer's progressed.

DN: I remember our meandering walk along the tropical pathways of your community. The picture you portray of this morning sounds healing and integrative, a new beginning.

IR: Yes, it is wonderfully tropical, and definitely a healing place. Now I live next to my favorite tree. I was elated to find this new place and actually proud to take the risk of moving as the COVID pandemic was beginning. I was on my own. I felt isolated and alone. I didn't ask anyone to help me move because COVID restrictions were so strict in this aging condo community and people around me were scared.

Still, I knew that moving was right. I relocated very slowly—carried three or four boxes to my second-floor unit every day; I counted the steps—14 steps to be exact—and walked very slowly carrying one box at a time, being very conscious of where I was putting my foot, so that I wouldn't fall. It took me two months.

Stairs were such an issue when I was taking care of Hal. I was terrified that he might lose his balance and fall down the stairs.

DN: As you were speaking, the image of the 14 steps up to your new home felt to me like a mirror image to Alzheimer's decline. One progress is up and the other is down, but moreover, going up you could count to 14 and anticipate arriving at your new home doorstep, while Alzheimer's end is not predictable.

IR: Dorit, this is an interesting reflection—one that I will dwell on. My journey with Alzheimer's decline did not feel like a downward process but rather a process of being there for him as he was losing his abilities, one bit at a time. I used to say that when, yet another function disappeared, one more lightbulb had burned out. That helped me to understand a bit of what was going on with him and to better accept his deterioration.

DN: Hearing your characterization of your relationship with Hal during his decline as "being there for him" rather than going downward is so helpful. It clarifies for me how my assumptions about the experience of being present to a loved one during a long-term, degenerative disease shaped the images that came up for me in response to your sharing.

I realize that I entered our conversation carrying my own experiences of sudden loss, and that they've colored my perception of you. I also imagined, as you spoke, carrying those boxes up the steps, as if you could finally contain your belongings; some I imagined holding memories from your life with Hal. And that containment and sure step could feel like such an opposite to how difficult it must have been to contain your anticipatory grief. But there again, is this my projection?

IR: Dorit, I don't think that I was trying to contain my anticipatory grief but rather navigate through it in a healthy way. I have learned to experience this grief as a natural expression of love. Walking up those stairs with heavy boxes was more like climbing the metaphorical mountain—trying to get to the other side of Alzheimer's and beginning in a new place with a new reality. It felt like an empowerment process that required courage and strength.

DN: Thank you so much for taking the time to describe the many layers of your experience so I can distinguish it from what the steps image brought up in me. Was your process gradual? Has Hal's gradual progress through Alzheimer's provided you time to gain this deeper understanding and nuanced awareness?

IR: Right, the ending of Alzheimer's is long; in fact, it is often referred to as "the long goodbye." And that really describes it well. So, I persevered—one day at a time, one step at a time, not knowing how long this journey would be as I watched his decline, holding on to each moment. It was very difficult, very trying. My desire was simply to be present to him in the moment while I was experiencing so much anticipatory grief. I feel very emotional as I share this.

DN: Thank you for being so open in describing your experience. It is a gift to hear you share this. I know it is your journey, but your process through it feels like a teaching.

IR: Yes. It was a teaching for me as well. For example, when Hal was placed in a home, I experienced, to my surprise, a letting go—a letting go of some of the stress, some of the grief, and a lot of the responsibility. I didn't expect this response. I now had a team that supported Hal's journey and I very much felt supported by this team. I now knew that I didn't have to do it all myself.

DN: I wonder whether the publication of your memoir and perhaps the intention of this conversation to share your grieving experience with others feel like an extension of being supported by others while Hal was still with you? It seems to me that by sharing your story, you might lend support to those who relate to your journey.

IR: Yes, the story was written to support people on similar journeys. Readers are invited to hold a very difficult story, although my intention at the time was to share moments that transcended the difficult Alzheimer's experience and showed that there could still be a loving relationship even as someone is losing his abilities. I felt very called to write this story and I wrote every night at two a.m.

DN: I'm deeply moved and intrigued by how your depiction of this spring morning in your new Florida home has led us into some recollections of your life with Hal. Imagery can be very powerful that way. I'd like to retrace back to where we started and tell you about today here in New York, and let's see where it takes us... It's a cloudy day here too, but the air is warming; we're going to have a nice, warm day tomorrow, like the mid-50s. The snowdrops are already opening; the daffodils are poking up. So spring is emerging. I remember that you mentioned how you thought of your creative expression and the many other transformative experiences you had in the process of grieving as transitioning from winter to spring. So I love that our conversation is taking place in spring, with all the signs of opening to new growth.

I wonder if my description of this forthcoming spring renewal is transporting you back to your years in upstate New York, at your home in the woods in Willow? All of a sudden, I'm really aware of the history of our relationship, and remembering Hal 17 years ago, before his diagnosis...

Can we each take a few minutes now to draw whatever emerges from our current inner landscapes? You had this idea that we could take our inspiration from the artwork on your book cover, and I liked it, because your painting of Hal and you embracing by the bay at sunset, with the heron by your side, has truly transported me into your world as I began reading your memoir. I wonder what will emerge for us now.

[conversation pauses for the drawing process]

DN: Can I share with you what I drew? [holding drawing to the screen]

IR: I see those feathers and the heron.

DN: Three feathers: messengers of gifts along the way. I began by entering the world of your painting and resonating with it, but then it seemed like your image was changing. In my drawing, the sunset is turning into a sunrise, and the heron, who was sitting still next to Hal and you, has spread its wings on the horizon. Looking at it now, the heron looks all-embracing and protective.

IR: It's so interesting; I have three feathers on my altar. They represent the whole journey. This feels like a synchronicity.

DN: Yes. And I associate three with synthesis and integration... Would you like to share your drawing with me?

IR: I made three drawings! This one [agitated line drawing in blue marker] feels like the inside of me right now, kind of wired-up thinking about all that is going on in Ukraine; I am so sad about what's going on in the world right now, and terrified—more sad than anything. I feel great heaviness in my heart. It feels like the world's grief is playing into my personal grief.

My second drawing reflects the sun. Is it a sunset or a sunrise? Perhaps both. Perhaps the journey went from sunset to sunrise.

And the last image are daffodils—I believe that they reflect the stage of "winter into spring," a new beginning.

DN: It seems like your three drawings are taking you full circle, from being present to your felt senses right now, to the echoes of grief in the world in your own journey of grief, and back to the present moment and your hope for a new beginning...

IR: In a funny sort of way.

DN: I wonder where it takes us now in our process? It feels like these drawings brought us to being really present to each other... We had a plan for this project and thought ahead about purpose and structure, and all of a sudden it feels like we're really here, in our hearts, with what's happening today, in nature around us, with our families, but also out there in the world. It's so interesting how all these worlds, past and present, far away and nearby, are never disconnected. And we're always in transformation.

I am reminded of my work with clients in art therapy; how I never know what might unfold in the hour we spend together and have to trust in the synchronicities and the wisdom of how everything eventually gets interwoven if we are willing to shine the light into that inner world.

It feels like you and I have begun our weaving of a new, ever-expanding narrative.

Earlier in our conversation, you spoke about your journey with Hal unfolding moment to moment with so much unknown, all so unpredictable, despite a definite prognosis. And I was thinking how challenging it must have been to remain present, especially because you don't know what will happen next, when it's going to end. And if you assume that it is going to go on for a long time, you might miss all these precious moments, like your light hearts and moments of laughter, which stayed with me from my visit to your home.

IR: The truth is that I didn't focus on the prognosis as much as on the quality of our relationship. We knew what it was, and we knew where it started and, of course, we found support. It was more important for me to try to be there for him. And it was not always easy. As I let go of expectation and anticipation of anything predictable, I let go of having to make sense of what he was saying, and just took him for who he was in the moment, and it became easier.

My experience as a transpersonal expressive arts therapist and educator was very helpful as I navigated these waters. I had experience with following the lead of what was happening in the moment, intuitive ways of understanding circumstances, and had cultivated deeper levels of listening through my life's work. That all helped me to navigate Alzheimer's and all of the strangeness of the illness with greater ease.

In the world of creative exploration and expressive arts, we often engage in imaginal realms and are deeply aware of metaphors. In a funny way, communicating with Hal was easier if I just listened to what he was saying through the lens of metaphor and imagination. Then we could enjoy one another and laugh a bit more.

In my experience with Hal, I found that just going with *his* reality and following his lead took the pressure off of him and off of me. And it added to our ability to relate to one another, to be in the moment and for me to be present to him. It was a way of honoring him.

DN: In a way, that was truly accepting him, sometimes in a playful way, joining him in his world and staying together on his terms rather than trying to pull him back to your reality. And isn't that what we do in our creative process? We are willing to venture into an imaginal realm and let it guide us into unconditional acceptance.

IR: Such a good point. Being in a relationship with someone who has Alzheimer's could very well be a creative process, if we let it be. Like in creative exploration, we follow the flow to see where an idea or image leads. Living in a relationship with someone who had Alzheimer's was similar to this for me. I never knew what would happen next. I stayed open to curiosity.

For example, there is a chapter in my memoir—"It's You! Yes! But Who Am I?"—where I share my realization that he didn't really know who I was or that I was his wife. That was OK. He identified me as his best girlfriend. Accepting this allowed us to enjoy one another because we simply played, danced, sang together. It really didn't matter that he didn't know my name or our relationship.

DN: I think that's where compassion is—being there unconditionally, with feeling. Not asserting yourself, imposing your reality, leading the way. I find this conversation brings tremendous compassion within me, being with you and listening, but I'm also aware of projecting my own stories of grief as I respond to your reflection.

IR: Compassion was an interesting thing, and it wasn't automatic during difficult moments. I ended up creating a mantra for myself that helped me to live my life and to make decisions with proper discernment. My mantra was: "Is this compassionate to him? Is this compassionate for me?" If I could say "yes" to both questions, then I would proceed. As an example, I made a decision *not* to visit him in his home every day. I decided to visit him three or four days a week for one or two hours at a time. This was a compassionate decision for both of us. It created a space for both of us to develop community in our new lives. It freed us from dependency and created healthy boundaries within a very difficult situation.

DN: It sounds like you're describing a healing container in this mantra, a container for dismantling the old narrative and creating a new one. Your mantra "compassionate for him and compassionate for me" seems to be a cognitive container for both Hal and your own self-care. Then the stories you co-created within this shared reality could be imaginal and playful.

IR: I appreciate the notion of "cognitive container." I needed a container for this experience in order to be grounded. Heartwood Manor [not the real name], the home where Hal was placed, was a container as well. It supported his everyday needs and freed me to have my own life, and more importantly to be present to him in loving ways.

Right before he moved to his new home, life was filled with so much grief, so much stress, and so much hypervigilance. Stress and hypervigilance are killers, and there were moments when I realized that I could very well die. My body was beginning to feel the toll of the stress, and each night I wondered if this was the day that I would die.

It turned out that placement was, in fact, really good for him. Heartwood Manor was surrounded by nature in a very beautiful setting with a pond, which was what he cared about more than anything. This living situation met his need for support, beauty, and community.

Again, my life's work taught me to listen deeply to the needs of my clients and students without overly directing and to flow with what was emerging in the moment and allowing it to reveal itself in a safe environment. This prepared me for being present to Hal.

My work also taught me to experience and move through what was emotionally emerging within me as well and to find ways to transform these feelings.

DN: It seems to me that being in nature was yet another container for you and Hal. It was a new ground for meeting each other differently. The natural world met you too, in some mystical ways.

IR: Yes! Nature provides much inspiration for living. It grounds, heals the heart, and provides so many opportunities for awareness through synchronicity. I had learned to pay attention to synchronicities, and I often experienced these within the natural world.

Here's an example.

One day a large flock of great white ibis (I call them great white herons in my book) flew over the pond at Heartwood Manor. I was intrigued because I had recently found an ibis feather on top of my purse in a screened-in bar.

I had no idea how it got there, and no one claimed it as their own. I took note and took the feather home. The ibis flock and the single feather felt like waking dreams. I just paid attention.

Soon after that, I had a dream about a house being built that had two bedrooms. I was deciding which room to claim as my own. One bedroom had a fireplace on the outside of the house and the other had very large windows. Through the window, I could see a large heron. It was looking into the window. This room was clearly the more desirable of the two. I wrote this dream down.

A few weeks later, the owners of Heartwood Manor announced that they were closing the home. This was devastating at this stage of Alzheimer's. I now had to do the hard work of finding another place for Hal and visited two different homes. The first placement, chosen by the Heartwood Manor owners, was a traditional memory care unit; the second, the Weaver House, was a small dwelling where a couple took care of four people. I wasn't sure what to do until the heron arrived.

As I visited Weaver House, I noticed a statue of a heron on the property. I asked about this. The owner informed me that there was a "beggar" heron that would come to the feeder. She showed me a photo of one of the residents who was feeding this large bird from her hand. I then remembered my dream and knew immediately that this is where I would place Hal, and I did. He transitioned three weeks later. He was well taken care of, and it was the perfect place for him to die.

DN: It sounds like it was also a beautiful place for closure, for you to say goodbye to Hal. As I've been listening, I found myself following the thread in your narrative, suspending the need to know how it was going to end up, despite knowing the inevitable. And I hear you saying that at some point you were also in a place of having released that need to figure it out ahead of time; you followed your heart, the signs in your dreams, and their synchronicities in waking life.

IR: Yes, I felt my way through this experience and, definitely, my spirituality taught me to pay attention to my intuition, which included synchronicity.

Creative Nonfiction and Transformative Grief
DN: I am so captivated by your process. It seems as if after Hal died, and

you have said your goodbyes, you could finally begin to retrace and revisit your story in a new way, threading the connections. The connections were made moment to moment, but the thread that was linking them together was truly visible in your memoir, in a way that contained and integrated the whole of your journey.

When I read your book, I was really moved by your celebration of life, unvarnished. It was uplifting, especially what felt like to me your connection with nature as a messenger of Spirit. Alzheimer's is associated with forgetting, and what you have done seems to be all about remembering, remembering to live, to laugh, to remain tender.

I also want to say that one of the things that left a deep impression on me is how your creativity comes through in writing your memoir, but it seems like your lifelong spiritual attunement prepared you long before your writing ensued, to pause and pay attention to synchronicities, trust your intuition, not only make rational decisions or what makes sense logically. You really felt your way through this whole journey.

IR: Yes, my memoir was also a creative process, and as is usual for me, it was accompanied by intuition and dream life. I knew I would write a book about the sacred moments that can emerge during Alzheimer's after an experience that opened my heart after a long, trying day of caregiving. This thought sat on the back shelf until after Hal's death. Then, one night, I had a dream. In that dream, the muse arrived and told me that it was time to write my book proposal. So I did! I always listen to my dreams.

My memoir actually looked very different from the original proposal, while retaining its essence. The proposal morphed from a spiritual self-help book into a memoir, also guided by my dreams. My experiences wanted to come through as a story. Ultimately, I discovered that I could share my awareness more fully through story.

Dreams and songs came nightly in my sleep, and these would inform me what chapters I would write at two o'clock each morning. That is when the muse arrived, and I couldn't miss a date with that muse! I followed the thread that was emerging and started writing from the insight of my dreams.

For example, one night I woke up singing "White Rabbit," and I thought about the words from *Alice in Wonderland*: "curiouser and curiouser." Suddenly, I was writing about the place where Hal was living, where things were getting curiouser and curiouser, where the residents were often in their own realities.

During these wee hours of the night, I would write until the writing felt complete and then go back to bed. I followed what was emerging without controlling it; I fully trusted the process. I learned that from Natalie Rogers. She would tell us to put our creative exploration by our beds, and when we woke up in the morning, notice what it was saying to us. I've been doing that with myself and others for a long time, and now this practice informed my creative writing process.

Painting the Way Through Grief

DN: I want to turn to the artworks you shared in your memoir. When we began the interview, you mentioned how your typical form of expression is immediate, like the quick drawings we each made today, flowing and outpouring intuitively. But the paintings you made in the process of grieving took a while to complete. You really took weeks to tune in to what they needed to become and layer colors and elements over time.

Can you share about what brought you to painting during your grieving process? My impression is that your paintings were integral to processing your anticipatory grief and also carried you through following Hal's death.

IR: Yes, they carried me in tender moments. The painting during this time emerged in an art class. As a creative arts therapist, I often created and asked my clients to express themselves within short periods of time and then talk about what was emerging for them in the moment. It is a relatively quick process that is connected to insight.

While I did use sandplay, images, authentic movement, and other forms of expression to process grief with my therapist, I also found that on my own, I spent longer periods of time painting and writing. As the grieving process intensified, I found myself doing art that reflected my anticipatory grief, and it took weeks and months to complete. Before Hal died, I worked on two pieces that felt like a lovers' embrace.

I had just asked him the question "How will I know it's you when you're gone?" I didn't want Hal to leave without us having a plan. Hal's favorite color was blue, so we kind of decided he would come back to me as a bluebird. The art teacher respected my process. She saw my tenderness and the tenderness in the lovebirds in the middle of the Triptych.

The picture on the front cover of my book emerged from a workshop on painting sunsets. I went there specifically to learn to paint sunsets, but suddenly other images began to form, and I simply paid attention. Hal and I appeared in my painting, and suddenly, a heron materialized, and then cranes, who were actually angels, emerged in my imagination and then onto the painting. The sunset shifted from a straight line to an image of light that was taking Hal into the heavens. Later, I recognized this image as telling the story of our relationship through the Alzheimer's journey from marriage into death.

One night, I woke up from my sleep and heard the words: "Finish it, frame it, and get it to Hal today." So I put the final touches on it, framed it, and hung it in the bedroom where he was being cared for. He exclaimed with wide eyes and said, "This is BEAUTIFUL!" (I wondered if he was referring to the image or the dying process reflected in the image.) The next day he lost his ability to speak or stand. He became bedridden and died a few days later.

After Hal died, I continued to paint as I grieved his actual death. Each painting took months and, again, came through songs that were playing in my head. They reflected the grieving stage that I was experiencing.

The first painting after Hal died reflected a deep feeling of loss. I called it "Crying to the Moon," a take-off on Bruno Mars' song "Talking to the Moon." In the song, he sings about sadness and solitude after a loss of someone he wants back.

The second painting, which I call "Meanwhile Life Goes On," was inspired by a line from Mary Oliver's poem "Wild Geese." This was a time in my grieving process where I felt numb—somewhat frozen—even as life was beginning to open more fully to me. I knew that eventually the grief would subside; life was happening around me, and yet I still felt disconnection from it all. This stage lasted a very long time, and I kept hoping that it would be over soon. I painted on this image until I finally felt an emergence of the possibility of a new day.

The last painting, which I call "It's a New Day," began to viscerally reveal itself. It came through an awareness of a movement. I saw this movement, I felt this movement, I drew this movement of clicking heels, and then later on, as I was watching the movie *Eat, Pray, Love*, I noticed a scene where Julia Roberts is in Bali, and she finally allows herself to experience love. As she walks away from her beloved, she clicks her heels together. I thought, "Oh my God, there it is—it's a new day." That's a wonderful archetypal image for a new day. I haven't framed this painting yet. Perhaps the new day is continuing to emerge.

Right now, I am looking at the image of the daffodils that I made at the beginning of this interview, and I'm feeling like this, too, is part of that energy of the new day. It's not quite there yet. I wrote the word "transition" in this first drawing with the sun. I had a sense of sunrise, but it really was both a sunset and sunrise. Those of us who work with creative exploration, no doubt, have similar understandings about how images reflect inner states.

Closure

DN: I'm so moved by the many forms of creative expression you've reached for that ushered you through your anticipatory grief and deep sadness for Hal's loss. It seems like your lifelong immersion in intuitive painting, authentic movement, listening to your dreams, paying attention to synchronicities, and following your felt sense guided this process. The beauty of imagery is that it activates all the senses, and anything is possible in our imagination and artwork, even clicking your heels when your body can no longer do that [smile].

I never thought before our conversation that grieving could become a creative process. But I guess death and dying are aspects of life; and living is a creative process, if we know how to see it that way, especially amid the challenges of caregiving.

I think you were positioned in a very unique way to discover, during your 11 years with Hal following his Alzheimer's diagnosis, how this "long goodbye" can be creative, expressive, and tender. I believe that others who walk these types of long grieving journeys with so much unknown, and the counselors who support them, would appreciate your insight.

IR: I do hear from people who read my book, and who have gone through similar circumstances. They say something like "Your story has helped me so much; I'm not afraid to read your story. It does not frighten me like many other books on Alzheimer's do."

DN: I wonder if it is also the love and self-care that permeate your memoir that help others move through their grief rather than sink back into the loss. As art therapists, too, when we facilitate a creative process, we want it to not be re-traumatizing. It must be safe to enter the process despite the grief and sadness it evokes. We must convey the feeling that creative expression is healing.

IR: I think that's why subconsciously I knew to change my original idea for a book into a memoir. Story is a powerful creative form that leads with the heart. It heals.

People have asked if writing my book was cathartic. I don't think it was, I think I simply had to write the story. It no longer feels like my story, even though it is. It was just a story that needed to be shared.

DN: I am grateful for the opportunity to join you as you encircled your journey once more today. It felt like, together, we gained some new insight and uncovered new layers of meaning. It felt healing to me.

IR: Thank you for interviewing me, Dorit.

I am aware that my heart feels heavy. I think it reflects both the re-emergence of grief over Hal's death, and also because of the state of the world right now. So many people are in deep grief for their homeland, as well as their family. All that is sparking my own grief and I don't even know how to help.

DN: Yes, I hear you. It's like another dimension of resonance with grief and the feeling of helplessness. We can't help but feel the reverberation of what's happening in Ukraine, and there's no way to contain that.

IR: Somehow there's got to be a way, even if it's simply through prayer.

Grief and Healing Through Creative Expression

At the outset of this interview, I was aware of my own experiences of loss: loss of childhood, loss of homeland, loss of my younger sister to cancer—losses I still carry with me. I wasn't sure how it would be for me to witness Ilana's process of reflecting on her grief, and what it would be like to resonate with her through the lenses of my own experience. My interest in this form of co-creative conversation is very much linked to my work as a creative art therapist. In art therapy, regardless of our expertise, we often begin with an empty page, perhaps with silence, but the page is never truly blank, and our minds are rarely quiet. We create a safe space, however, to look at this empty container to be filled—filled with images that reflect our lived experiences, memories, feelings, core beliefs, and signs of open wounds that long to heal.

The intention of my conversation with Ilana was, similarly, to provide a safe container for her reflections about her journey, this time with me as a witness.

In her memoir, Ilana wrote about how her stories reflected moments that sustained and taught her something important about compassion, kindness, renewal, acceptance, and patience, making difficult decisions, arriving at a balance between caring for her husband and self-care, and discovering deeper levels of meaning (Rowe, 2020). In our interview, too, there were threads that together seem to have intuitively weaved Ilana's narrative in ways that transcended the arduous, at times frustrating, and progressively challenging role of caring for Hal as his Alzheimer's symptoms advanced.

Shortly after I read the interview transcript, I came across the writing of Kathryn Schultz. The following reflection Schultz provided on loss and love seemed to encapsulate the quality of tenderness preserved in Ilana's journey, despite the hardship and through her grief:

> If we are lucky enough, if we are stubborn enough, we love and we lose and then the loss opens us up to more love—different love, because each love is unrepeatable and irreplaceable—on the other side of grief; love unimaginable from the barren landmass of loss, love without which, once found, the world comes to feel unimaginable. (Schultz, 2022)

I experience personal stories as images that activate all the senses in their recollection, in listening, and in the process of shared meaning making. Ilana spoke of dreams, music, song lyrics, and poems, serendipitous moments, signs given to her in nature, and art making. There was a quality of looking back and noticing how her stories evolved through the stages of Alzheimer's toward and beyond Hal's death. But what was most palpable to me is how these expressive ways of being and relating seem to have emerged moment to moment and kept her moving (authentically), vital, loving, and even joyful amid the everyday routines as well as twists and turns on a winding road many would lamentably describe as going downhill.

As we began the interview with our quick drawings, I was lost in the moment, listening and taking in Ilana's artwork and reflections. But at the end, I was surprised by the feeling the interview left within me. Despite the heaviness of suffering that was broadcasted across the ocean from Ukraine, which colored our thoughts, Ilana's story of her creative journey through

Alzheimer's was uplifting, a spiritual teaching. We noticed signs of spring in our gardens, but also felt that transition of winter into spring in our conversation, with hope for a new day, with a prayer. Our dialogue validated something I already knew but did not realize I brought with me to the blank page of our conversation—the sense of living life as a creative process no matter what.

As I revisited the questions I had in the beginning—What will we gain and lose in this process? Will it connect us more deeply with life and with those we each lost? Will it prepare us further for our continued life journeys and for that which remains a mystery? What might emerge through our collaboration that could not have transpired without it?—I gained deeper appreciation for the gift of being entrusted to listen to another person's story; a shift in my view of anticipatory grief and the role of creative expression in the process of grieving; an affirmation of the power of intuition to guide us in our daily lives and in art making when faced with the unknown.

With gratitude for our collaboration and the opportunity to examine my assumptions about anticipatory grief, I reached out to Ilana and asked her about her thoughts following our conversation. In turn, she thanked me for the opportunity to explore more fully her creative expression in response to anticipatory grief. She wrote:

> This dialectic interview process has truly been rewarding and a learning experience. It has helped me to better understand and articulate my personal story and brought me to new awareness. My greatest take-away from this interview was a deepening appreciation of how potent creativity can be in our lives if we listen to what is emerging. Living a creative lifestyle enlightens all that we do and is inseparable from who we are. In my story, creativity became part of my caregiving, self-care, and my grieving process. The imagination is food for the soul, a nourishing and transformative energy that informs our insights if we listen to what is emerging. It can make hard times easier to digest and sometimes even playful. It can soothe our heartaches and help us to become more whole.

It follows that part of our role as educator or therapist is to support others as they cultivate their own creative and intuitive ways. Creative expression is certainly a healing modality—expressive arts therapists already know this.

Shifting creative exploration from technique to a natural way of being in the world can unleash the healing powers of creative expression as we walk through life.

References

Anderson, R. & Braud, W. (2011). *Transforming Self and Other Through Research: Transpersonal Research Methods and Skills for the Human Sciences and the Humanities*. State University of New York Press.

Creswell, J.W. & Miller, D.L. (2000). Determining validity in qualitative inquiry. *Theory into Practice, 39*(3), 124–130. http://dx.doi.org/10.1207/s15430421tip3903_2

Ferrer, J.N. (2011). Participatory spirituality and transpersonal theory: A ten-year retrospective. *The Journal of Transpersonal Psychology, 43*(1), 1–34.

May, R. (1994). *The Courage to Create*. Norton. (Originally published 1975.)

Netzer, D. (2016). Transpersonal art: Conversation with artist Judy Schavrien. *Art/Research International Journal, 1*(1), 211–214. doi:10.1177/1077800414566686

Netzer, D. (2017). Passage: A conversation with Jill Mellick. *The Journal of Transpersonal Psychology, 49*(2), 124–130. doi:10.1207/s15430421tip3903_2

Roulston, K. (2010). *Reflective Interviewing: A Guide to Theory and Practice*. Sage.

Rowe, N.I. (2020). *Sacred Stories: A Caregiver's Journey Through Alzheimer's*. Independently published.

Schultz, K. (2022). *Lost and Found: A Memoir*. Random House.

Way, A., Zwier, R.K. & Tracy, S.J. (2015). Dialogic interviewing and flickers of transformation: An examination and delineation of interactional strategies that promote participant self-reflexivity. *Qualitative Inquiry, 21*(8), 720–731. doi:10.1177/1077800414566686

CHAPTER 12

Creating Meaning Through Nature

Louise Allen

Introduction

Although we may feel stuck at points, we are always moving in some way. We, in and of nature, are continually transitioning. Whether that's the flow of our breath, the ageing of our bodies, the changing of our thoughts, or the seasons shifting around us; the smells and sounds and sights we receive continually flowing. One pattern of both shape and movement that I observe in nature is spirals—both as a noun and a verb. From flower buds and ferns that coil themselves tightly when it's dark and unfurl and bask in the light. To snail shells that spiral and protect, that enable the mollusc to reach out when it is safe to do so and retract when there is a threat.

For me, spring, with its abundance of emerging and opening (and where I am in the UK, sometimes retreating when it gets frosty again), is one of the most visible teachers of this process. There is something repetitive, continual, consistent and evolutionary in this. How we relate to the spiralling varies greatly from person to person. Perhaps it is reassuring that night follows day follows night. That spring will follow winter. Perhaps it is stifling or feels restrictive. Perhaps it is a blend of emotions dependent on our inner and outer situations and conditions.

Spirals remind me of our inner processes. In the way we can make ourselves smaller, or not share our feelings or thoughts, beliefs and desires, or act in a way that doesn't feel comfortable. Coiling ourselves up tightly for a whole multitude of reasons. And how there is an inner part of us often also wanting to spread out, to be seen as we are and grow into our fullest potential. How we can sometimes feel the need to open up and share everything, and what that then means for the vulnerable part of us that needs to curl back in sometimes.

There is often something concentric and layered, for example in seeds, nuts and flowers. Their different qualities allow freedom of movement (by wind, animal, momentum) and safety until they are ready to open and risk exposing a more tender, vulnerable interior (hard shells, tight pods, prickles). I also think of labyrinths, symbols humans have created for hundreds of years across the world. A continual path in and out, space to pause in the centre, and then make our way back out again. Then there are tides, our breath, ripples, mandalas, in and out, to and fro, ebb and flow. These natural movements, which we are part of in the physical dimension of our experience, chime for me with our psychological experience captured in the dual process model of grief. The idea that we need both to be with our loss, and to be with the creation of something new, of restoring life. And that we move between the two processes at our own pace. I think both processes can feel both closed and open, too.

I recently walked in a new-to-me area of the South Downs and was struck by pine trees I had not seen before. From a distance, I saw the shape of draped branches. Closer up, these branches appeared to be dripping with tiny tuft-shaped clusters of needles and small, round pine cones. After stumbling through churned and dried mud and browned, brackeny thicket—reminders of the preceding wetter, darker months—to get a closer look still, I realised that the needles weren't in fact hard spikes as I had imagined, but soft and feathery. As I reflect on that walk a few weeks later, I notice the curiosity that drew me on and out; a link between the trees and something within me. Later that evening, I identified the tree as a larch, a deciduous tree that loses its needles in the winter. Nature's reminder that what at first appears threatening or hostile is often a signal to something softer and vulnerable. Not knowing the name of the tree hadn't detracted from my wonder and appreciation of what I saw and discovered; the shapes and patterns of something not before known drew me in. My continued wondering then led me to find out more and make sense of what I had seen, identifying the tree and learning a little about the life cycle of the larch.

While connecting our feelings, the way we relate with others and our experiences can be an enlightening and freeing part of the therapeutic process, making sense of and understanding why and how we experience the world as we do. Being with the unknown and its nonsensicalness is also something that resonates with my approach to therapy; we may not be able to always rationalise, make sense of or identify a sense or emotion we experience. But we can still get to know that experience as it is and find a way to make meaning. Working creatively when we don't have the words to convey our experience can be a powerful way of connecting to our inner world and with others. It just might open up a new way of understanding our life.

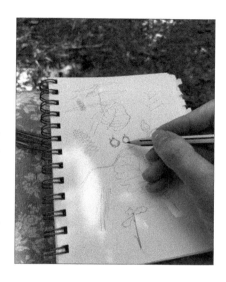

Whether we understand the whys and hows of nature, nature continues regardless with her patterns, shapes and processes. Embracing what we observe and are drawn to in nature when we don't know what to say, or can't make sense of where we are at, can enable something new to emerge. We might be led by a search for meaning, or from an inner curiosity. We might be led by nostalgic memories, or we may begin from engaging our senses and let the world around us lead.

The following is a reflection of one woman's experience of engaging with nature-inspired asemic writing. Asemic writing is a visual art form suggesting symbols, words or letters but without semantic meaning. Devoid of a mutually understood language, asemic poetry, like abstract art, allows for the "reader" to interpret the meaning. Her words are used with her permission.

> I had been drawn to this work, exploring transitions, as a significant change in my life has brought me intense grief and uncertainty this year. I was interested in working with Louise in nature, as I lean heavily on my connection to the earth as a way of sustaining myself day to day... We met at a local woodland early in the evening... I felt great relief to walk deeper into the wood and away from the sounds of the road that I find very difficult to tune out.
>
> I was drawn to this mature beech tree... I loved this tree, for its beauty and strength standing tall with multiple bifurcated trunks standing together as one. Its bright and deep litter carpeted the ground in a circle at its feet, and

whilst this litter had stopped other plants growing there, I really felt invited in. The canopy it had formed created a dome-like green roof over the space and I felt it offered us protection from the rain that was really beginning to fall. I felt really enclosed.

We sat down on coats and blankets on the wet floor, and I was invited to draw something of interest to me here. With the rain, the earth felt really connected to the sky that was crying! I started by drawing just the skeleton of the bifurcating branches above as their pattern and form really appealed to me. The rain was falling heavily, and I thought my precious paper that I'd kept for something special was disintegrating. Louise felt that it was significant that I'd let myself bring this treasured paper "saved for a rainy day" to the session.

After I while, having lost sense of time, I asked Louise if I should stop. She introduced the idea of creating an asemic poem. I hadn't even heard this word before, and she described what it meant. It felt freeing to be invited to make something next that would have no specific meaning or semantic content. Although I didn't fully understand, I went with it and looked for the pieces or parts of my "alphabet" within the drawings and marks I'd just made. It was interesting and alarming to me that with the word "alphabet" in my mind, I immediately saw the letters FEA in my tree branch drawing. I couldn't look for an R but pulled from my work both these found letters and other shapes and forms that I was drawn to, to compile an alphabet of 12 "letters."

Louise encouraged me to make my poem, by reassembling them into a new piece of my choosing. I was unsure how to do this "right," and whilst it was made clear that there was no right or wrong, Louise supported me by showing me examples of how this could be done. I created a poem starting with the FEA letters that had jumped out at me. I then arranged parts of my alphabet in decreasing size and firmness. At the bottom of my curve outwards, I drew my forms very firmly—redrawing lines to make them very bold. I then repeated the F letter, and after this my poem closed with very lightly marked and smaller sweeping forms, drifting away to nothing.

Louise encouraged me to look at it from a different angle and to think about what I saw in it, perhaps searching for meaning there. I [saw] an energy in its curving form, making something like a wave, but then I thought of water, with my line work flowing like ripples on the surface of a river running. When I'd originally drawn the branch, I thought about a river form or veins—maybe blood running? I thought about the branching and twisting, moving river of my life as we touched on this. I noticed the crossing forms in the lines I had drawn and thought of two lives entwined.

I explained I'd been shocked in thinking my drawing had included the word FEAR in my first reading of potential letters there, but that I'd worked with this and cut off the word with new letters of my own making. A flurry of meaning sprang from the piece as I spoke about my fears at this juncture in my life.

I spoke of a determination and strength I'd recognised in myself earlier that day, finding my way in it all... In touching on these multi-layered parts of my poem, I really felt a strong wave of grief rush over me... Louise said that this grief was totally understandable in the context of all that was happening and allowed me to see this as natural as life chapters go. I did feel great relief as, together, we unpicked the marks I'd made... As I look on the piece again now, I can see so much in this strange poem.

I invited my client to return to the tree and reflect on why she had been drawn to it. She shared what she felt about the tree's skin and the strength and comfort it offered her. I called her attention to the surrounding holly which formed a ring around the stand of beech trees. My client felt that this created a "prickly protection" around the trees and spoke of how much she loved trees and their endurance. She felt very connected to the earth through this exercise.

We closed our session, and I reminded her to be gentle with herself upon her return home, which she did. That evening, she woke up in the middle of the night and had this insight:

I came across a beautiful piece of writing titled "Being the compost heap" and I remembered that Louise had talked on the relevance of a part of my path forward, centred upon my work composting. I said that sometimes it feels like the only thing I do that makes sense! She spoke of the death life cycling and its relevance in the threads of our conversations during the evening:

To birth a world born of new stories of love and hope and connection, we must first create space for the old stories to die. We must hospice them. We must hold them as they take their last breaths.

We must become the compost heap. (Philips, 2022)

As one person reflects on the process of their journey with this creative technique, we see an interconnected journey emerge. The physical walk and invitation to observe provides an opportunity to connect with the natural world. As the steps of the asemic poem creation continue, the other-than-human world they were drawn to is transformed into their own shapes. Together, with curiosity, we gently enquire into what they see in their creation, and as to any significance or meaning in the world around us to which they were drawn.

This creative exercise is inspired by an asemic poetry writing workshop I attended, facilitated by experimental poet Michał Kamil Piotrowski. I have adapted it as a way of connecting with the natural world around us—plants, animals and landscapes. The intervention centres around the idea of finding inspiration and patterns that we are drawn to and opening them up, dismantling what we see and creating something new. I view this process as a collaboration between ourselves and other-than-human nature.

The following is inspired by and shared with kind permission from Michał Kamil Piotrowski.

Method

This exercise invites the creation of a new "alphabet" found in the shapes and patterns in nature. This new, unique alphabet is then used to create a visual poem or letter. The creative process incorporates mindfulness, observation of the natural world and receiving the natural world as inspiration to find shapes and patterns.

To begin with, the person is invited to create an asemic poem using their alphabet. Asemic means without meaning; and so we are creating something visual with a vacuum of meaning. The idea of asemic poetry is that it does not contain semantic meaning; it is devoid of a mutually understood language but may look like symbols, words or letters. Asemic poetry, like abstract art, is left for the "reader" to interpret and find their own meaning.

In the final stage of this process, the person becomes the "reader," filling in the absence of meaning with their own interpretation of what they have created.

It is important when working creatively that we do not touch someone's artwork/creative work unless they ask us to, or with their consent. You are inviting them to create something that is, or represents, a part of themselves and can quite quickly carry meaning and deep feeling.

Before using this intervention with anyone in a therapy session, ensure you have an idea of how long each stage might take so you can hold the time boundaries of the session and allow sufficient time for all stages to be completed. You might want to guide yourself through the stages and reflect on what comes up for you and how long you think is needed. From my experience, between one hour and 90 minutes is about right.

What You Will Need
- A pen/pencil and paper
- Other-than-human nature. This could be:
  - a natural environment (if working outdoors)
  - a selection of natural materials such as pine cones, plants, flowers, stones (if working indoors)
  - images of nature such as gardening or travel magazines or photos (if working indoors or online).

First

Introduce the intervention by explaining that you will be guiding them through the steps to create an asemic poem—a poem without meaning, but which looks as if it could be words on a page. As the aim is to create a poem without meaning, you will not ask them to think of a particular theme or topic. Instead, the creative process will allow for something to emerge.

You will be taking your inspiration from nature.

Take your pen/cil and paper and quickly sketch the lines and shapes of what you see. The aim is not to represent what you see perfectly, or even recognisably. It is to start identifying the shapes and lines of nature. This could be anything that intrigues you or that you notice.

It might include:

- the shape of petals
- a smaller aspect of something (e.g. bubbles of sea foam, or the shape of a moss flower)
- recurring patterns or shapes
- the spaces in between leaves/trees
- interesting marks on a stone

- the paths forged in the landscape
- silhouettes against the horizon.

You might want to turn the flowers/stones/pine cones around and see if you notice any shapes from a different angle. What does the tip of a stem look like? What shape is the side of a leaf?

Second
Take a second piece of paper.

This time, looking at what you have drawn in the first stage, pick out any interesting and simple shapes that you can see in your drawing. These should not be recognisable letters but may be shapes and lines which look as though they could be symbols or letters.

You might notice a particular swish of a line that you have drawn a few times, or a simple shape. There can be similarities, or they might all be wildly different. However, you should be able to distinguish one from another.

Draw these out. You can have as few or as many as you like, but bear in mind that these will form characters for your natural alphabet and you will use them to "write" during the next stage. Between three and 15 "nature characters" will enable flexibility in the next stage.

Third
Take a third piece of paper.

Using your natural alphabet, create a poem, write a letter or write a story.

Go with the flow—try to make it look like a poem, letter or story, but remember, it doesn't need to mean anything. You are visually representing what a poem, letter or story looks like.

Fourth
Explain that you would like to invite the person to bring themselves out of their creative process so that they take the position of "reader" of their creation rather than creator.

They might want to place their poem/letter/story somewhere they can see it from a different angle. Or switch seats.

They may also like to ground themselves in the space using the five senses exercise before continuing:

- Take three deep breaths.
- What are five things you see (out loud or in your mind)?
- What are four things you can touch/feel?
- What are three things you can hear?
- What are two things you can smell?
- What is one thing you can taste?

Fifth

Invite them to take the role of "reader" and share their observations using the following questions to guide your inquiry:

- What do you see?
- Tell me about anything that stands out.
- Do any aspects of the poem/letter/story remind you of anything?
- How does the piece make you feel?
- Is there a message in the poem? What do you think it is saying?
- Is there anything you would like to say to or do with the poem?
- Do any of these reflections have any significance for you in your own life?
- Is there anything else you would like to say?
- What will you do with the creation now?

Leave some time to close down the session and reflect on how they found the process.

How and When It Can Be Used

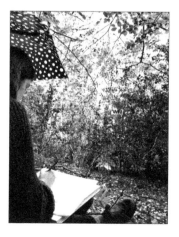

Although the creative process is facilitated, it is open to enable the person's individual creative process to emerge. Working in this way may be a helpful intervention if someone feels completely stuck, are unsure of how they feel or find they have no words or way "in" to their experience.

Inherently, the exercise is connective (with the natural world and the person's unconscious) and so might be helpful to someone feeling adrift and untethered in the wake of their loss. It may not bring about meaning making at this stage but facilitates a deeper and broader connection from which new possibilities for meaning may start to be explored and nurtured.

Once the person's "alphabet" is created, it enables a vast range of opportunities for using it beyond the session to communicate non-verbal messages. This might be about their experience, to someone who has died or they are no longer in contact with, to their future selves or anyone or anything else that they may want to explore communicating with.

Reference

Philips, H. (2022). Becoming the compost heap. Letters from Holiday, July 6. https://holiday.substack.com/p/becoming-the-compost-heap

There Was a Moment

There was a moment
as we were leaving the hospital room
when everyone else walked ahead.
I stopped,
took a step back,
leaned in,
just to check on him,
lying there,
alone,
waiting,
the late afternoon light
through the Venetian blinds
breaking in lines over him,
the television blinking with no sound,
his head turned slightly
to look at me
            around
          the corner
       of the doorway,
coming or going,
in an instant,
not knowing
at all
then
that
I should have stayed

~ Steven "Mud" Roues

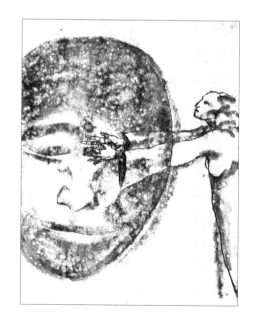

CHAPTER 13

The Rings of Identity
Exploring our Multiple Selves
Claudia Coenen

Our identity is challenged in grief. This feels disruptive and unsettling, as the world as we knew it seems lost to us. We expected that our lives would unfold in certain ways, and now our assumptions about how that will happen feel shattered. Bereavement includes rebuilding this sense of identity along with reconstructing the world in new ways so that we can live fully again after loss (Parkes, 2010).

Nothing made me more aware of the various parts of my Self than when I was suddenly shattered by the death of my husband, Alby, in the middle of our life together. I wrote about this feeling in my book *Shattered by Grief* (Coenen, 2018):

> [I]f my life was in pieces, I had to find a way to rebuild it. And it also occurred to me that I could, perhaps, rebuild it in a subtly new way. It was not as if I was suddenly going to become a doctor or move to Borneo. But if I was shattered, I might be able to take a closer look at all the broken shards of my Self and consider them. Maybe there were strengths, skills, attributes that I could enhance. Certainly there were character aspects I'd like to diminish a little, if I could not rid myself of them outright. So my sudden dance with Death did not have to mark the end of my life, although it was an end to my life as I knew it. Somewhere in the rubble, there were opportunities. Somewhere, inside the pain, so extreme it was almost physical, there had to be healing. Somehow, although I did not know how long it would take, I would find a way to grow from this calamity.

As unnerving as this loss of identity can be, it presents an opportunity to consider the multiplicity of Self. I have capitalized the S in Self to represent the whole Self, the actual unchangeable essence of our personhood, which contains all the different ways we manifest. We are complex beings, and our worldview is influenced by our thoughts, emotions and how we incorporate the philosophy of our family and culture as well as the choices we make to define our own way of being. We are also made up of who we are attached to, what we do, influenced by how and where we live. Adverse events can cause parts of us to congeal or hide, and yet there is an overarching integrity to the Self. We become aware of our wholeness when we experience moments of clarity and in times of peak experiences where rumination, pressures from societal expectations and other distractions fall away.

For me, finding my way back to a sense of integration and wholeness was compelling after I was bereaved. "Bereft" means to be deprived of something, which is how it feels when someone so close to you dies. The world seems to be missing its color, its shape. Some people even describe their loss as missing an arm or leg. Life does not feel normal, and many of the ways I defined myself seemed fragmented and no longer a part of me. My Self was cracked open.

How do we grapple with widowhood when we are used to defining ourselves as a spouse? When our parents die, are we orphans? Does that mean we no longer can define ourselves as someone's child? If our only child dies, are we still a parent? Since so many of our definitions of self are relational, the effects of death on who we are gives us pause.

We also define ourselves by what we do, our jobs and careers, our activities. Upon meeting someone new, we are often asked, "What do you do?" Since I don't believe what we do for money is the only viable part that represents us, I try to ask a different question. I might ask, "What are you engaged in?" or "Tell me something about your life." Yet what we do daily *is* part of who we are; this is how we present ourselves to the outer world.

By considering who and how we are in the world, in relationships and within ourselves, we can redefine our sense of self and rebuild our identity. We can begin by exploring different facets of what makes us who we are, including how we define ourselves and how we have changed by our connection to the person who has died.

My late husband, Alby, and I spent our early years attending weekend-long ceremonial workshops with a teacher named Elizabeth Cogburn. Elizabeth's work was grounded in ritual, stimulating deep inquiry into human nature, spirituality and right living (Cogburn, 1984). She invited us to explore conscious relationships. This was an interesting way to start a marriage and it informed ours from its beginnings in friendship, shifting into love, marriage and parenting. (As an aside, it is amusing to call Alby late as he almost always was.)

Elizabeth's gatherings were rooted in many traditions. Her early life included exposure to the Episcopal Church and Native American stories and traditions. Elizabeth was a social worker, a dancer and a student of Jean Houston's Mystery School and Dromenon, which explored ancient wisdom traditions. She was a student of the Builders of the Adytum (B.O.T.A.), a school of Qabbalah. Her "Long Dances" combined drumming, trance dancing and esoteric teachings (Koff-Chapin, 1983). Each weekend had a seasonal theme celebrating solstices, equinoxes and cross-quarter points of May Day, Lammas, Candlemas and All Hallows. There was a specific inquiry to focus on, and the gatherings began and ended with Talking Staff Circles, in which each person would have time to address the question. Elizabeth would hold aloft her medicine pipe as the Talking Staff, look around the circle of attendees and ask: "Do you love yourself enough to listen with the ears of your heart to the other voices of yourself speaking?"

This always struck me as a dual question. We were invited to pay close attention to what each person in the circle was saying, how they answered the inquiry and to open our hearts to hear them fully without judgment. The question evoked the idea of unity within the circle of participants, indicating that by gathering in community, we contributed our personal voices to the One Voice of the group. It also alluded to other voices of myself speaking, in my own interior world, in response to what others were saying.

Until recently, I believed this question was original to Elizabeth. But Deborah Koff-Chapin, who introduced us to Elizabeth years ago, told me that it was received in a dream by an early participant in Elizabeth's Long Dances, named Benno Kennedy. I am happy to attribute it correctly.

Who we are is formed by what we have been taught about how to live and interact with others. We absorb messages, encouragement and admonitions from parents and teachers as well as from events that shift our perspective. We live with a composite of these internal messages, and we develop our own as well. Sometimes, they seem like multiple voices within us. These are not literal voices but reminders of past influences, events and awareness of different aspects of self at different times in life. We recall past experiences which inform our current lives, coming to our assistance or standing in our way. Trauma can impede our development and our ability to succeed in some areas of our lives, but deep inner work on healing the wounded parts within us contributes to our personal growth. These messages and "voices" are available to inform us, and we also can listen to them or override them. If we are curious about the different parts of ourselves, we can view ourselves in our wholeness and incorporate these aspects as reminders and guides.

When I was a choreographer, I could call up the sensation in my mind and body of my younger self twirling and leaping as a child and use this as inspiration for my choreography. When we are about to do something that is challenging or new, we might hear a cautionary voice inside, warning us to be careful. After someone we care deeply about has died, we might experience what feels like their guidance from beyond.

It is common for people to say, "I don't know who I am anymore," since we tend to define ourselves in relation to others. Metaphors arise like "I've lost a piece of me" or "Half of my self is gone now." Some people find it hard to continue the work they did before their person died.

This question of loving myself enough to listen invites all the inner parts to join me and tell me what it is they want me to know. It also allows me, as the leader of this "group" if you will, to tell that one part that is particularly loud and intrusive to sit down for a while. Opening the ears of my heart to those other voices of my Self places *me* in a key position, allows me to be more amused than annoyed at the parts of myself that are getting in my way.

We are a compilation of the different selves we have been throughout our lives. We recognize this and express it when we say, "A part of me thinks this and another part feels this." What are these parts that make up who we are? To say it differently, *who* are these various "people" that live inside me, that attempt to protect me or make sure I don't embarrass myself or put myself in some danger? The younger parts of me have not really gone away; instead, they might arise in the form of my inner child who wants to play. There is an angry teen inside who believes she has been treated unjustly and has not been seen or supported for the talents she has. There is the part of me that is Before His Death and the part of me that struggled through widowing to become the part of me that is Now.

Who we are, or perhaps who we *think* we are, is often shattered by the disruption of death. I am aware that not everyone feels broken after someone dies, but many of us do. This breaking open is painful and disorienting. It also presents an opportunity for self-discovery, growth and reconstructing our lives to feel whole again.

These multiple selves are available to us, but they sometimes arise in unexpected ways. The part of us that is afraid to make a mistake or to be embarrassed by failure or exposure might be a useful reminder to be careful and consider options before making a move. But this may also hinder us from moving forward, if we follow that caution and don't ever take risks. Cultural anthropologist Angeles Arrien mentions that as we move towards a more integrated sense of self, hidden or "disowned" parts might arise and ask for attention. She says that as we become more comfortable in ourselves, we are "at home," but then those alienated parts come knocking (Arrien, 2008). This is similar to what Richard Schwartz (2021) refers to as our inner exiles, some of whom we may not be aware of.

The repair of my shattered self, of who I was before Alby died and who I have become since, has included parsing out various pieces of my identity in an effort to enter a dialog with those disowned, wounded parts, to operate more out of my own inner wise Self. Recognition of what has been broken or stunted and which parts are no longer serving the greater whole requires me to listen with the ears of my heart to these other voices. Once they are heard, they tend to settle down into the background which, in most cases, is where they belong.

Here are some common parts that arise in people.

The Inner Critic

Almost all of us have an Inner Critic, especially those of us who are creatives, and while the Critic may have some useful suggestions, more often than not my Inner Critic prevents me from following inspiration and keeps me from writing complete sentences. The more I try to ignore my Inner Critic, the louder she gets until I delete page after page or have to put down whatever I was trying to do and go take a walk. This, by the way, is a good way to circumvent the Critic; I imagine that I am taking her with me and will leave her sitting under a tree while I go back and start again.

The Inner Child

Recently, I went to brunch with Elizabeth Coplan, a dear friend and colleague, who is one of the writers in this book. The restaurant is decorated with old, rusted advertising signs from gas stations, pubs and pharmacies. My eye was drawn to a sign that was new. It stated, "All Adults Must be Accompanied by Their Inner Child at All Times."

When my son Eben was planning to propose to his girlfriend, he ventured into the desert on a Vision Quest. This was his third guided quest where he spent four days alone, without food, at a campsite of his own making. He had brought along basic camping essentials, the engagement ring and he also had with him, internally, his Inner Child. Eben describes his experience this way:

I chose to model my quest after the medicine wheel teachings we had discussed at length. Each shield is represented by a cardinal direction corresponding to a different stage of life, and with each direction comes the lessons of a season. South/Summer represents childhood and the lessons of trust and innocence, West/Fall represents adolescence and the lessons of introspection, North/Winter represents adulthood and the lessons of wisdom and the giveaway, and East/Spring represents birth/death and the lessons of the great mystery and the unknown.

After parting the group and entering into the sacred landscape where I would spend my next several days, I recounted other lessons we had discussed at basecamp. I found myself recalling a phrase we had discussed: "Medicine is anything that brings you closer to wholeness." I thought about this concept of wholeness, and the different parts of my own psyche. Before I let myself delve too deep, however, I remembered my intention for the day was to focus on the lessons of the South and childhood, so I decided to take a moment to address my inner child directly. Under the hot desert sun, I drew a line in the sand and spoke as a caring, loving adult to my younger self.

"Hello, I hope you're having a nice day. I was wondering if you wouldn't mind talking for a bit about these big new steps we are taking together?"

I paused for a moment, crossed to the other side of the line, and replied in the voice of my inner child, "Not really, that sounds boring. I would rather throw rocks."

And so, like a madman ranting alone in the wilderness, I reasoned with my inner child, listening to their needs, while also explaining what might be important to maintain balance going forward. A part of me was gripping to the past, not wanting to let go of my carefree lifestyle, to play, to be silly, and to not take anything too seriously. Yet there was another part of me that yearned for the next stages of life, marriage, children, a home to call our own, and I found at times these two sides jostled for power. My inner child wanted to ignore my responsibilities and focus on play, while my adult side knew we needed to shape things up and start taking steps towards a better future.

Sensing this dilemma, I struck a bargain with my inner child. I agreed that I would promise to set aside time to be goofy and to play, if they would help lend their exuberant energy to some of our more mundane tasks at home and work. This way, we could still honor each other's needs without shying away from the responsibilities of adulthood. Over the next several days, while I did spend many long hours engaged in meditation, I also made sure to honor the pact I made with my younger self. After a long period of reflection or ritual, I made sure to grant time to strip bare and dance across the hot sands like a desert creature. Careless, wild, feeling whole!

Eben has been able to dance with his Inner Child in the years since his Vision Quest and brings his sense of wonder, play and joy out to play with his own children.

Who I Am SUPPOSED to Be (Instead of Who I Really Am)

Our upbringing and the communities we live in influence how we conduct ourselves, what we decided to study and the careers we might engage in. Some educational systems track people, leading them towards certain outcomes, directing students either vocationally or professionally. Some parents expect their children to follow in their footsteps or insist that their child become a doctor or a lawyer instead of an artist out of fear that the creative path is not a lucrative one.

I attended a weekend workshop at Omega Institute with Richard Schwartz, the founder of Internal Family Systems (IFS) Theory (2021). He talked about the strong wishes of his father that he become a doctor and continue the family legacy. It took his father many years to see his accomplishments in the field of psychology and to recognize the contribution IFS has given to the understanding of the multiplicity of our selves.

People may choose a course of study and employment that is safe but does not challenge them or fulfill their sense of who they are. Some meet their life partners during their careers and, after the death of this partner, question whether they want to continue on this path. A client, a medical doctor, stopped practicing after the death of his husband of 32 years; he is uncertain what he will do next and questions whether he can define himself as a doctor if he has left the profession. I pointed out to him that not only was medicine what he did but being a person of healing is *who* he is. He now has an opportunity to use those skills and the qualities he brings to medicine in different ways; it just will take time to discover and develop what that will look like in his future.

Wounded Parts

We all have wounds, large and small. How we navigate the difficult times in our lives and how we grow through them influences how much these wounds might impede or encourage us. We may choose to isolate or exile these wounded parts of ourselves, hoping that by ignoring them we won't have to deal with the pain that part feels. Some people take this approach to their grief as well, pushing it aside or pretending that they are not affected by adopting a "stiff upper lip" manner, refusing to talk about the person who is gone or even to acknowledge that they are hurting. While this may work for a while, generally grief and pain will call out in some way for attention.

Allowing our wounded parts to inform us is often difficult as these hurt places react to current stimuli as if current events are splitting open old scars. It is important to remember that this is a feeling, albeit a strong one, and we can apply love and care to those old hurt places, recognizing the circumstances that caused them. We also can choose to soothe ourselves and let some of the old pain and anger go. There are many choices to be made with an old psychological or emotional hurt.

Engaging Inner Parts

There are other methods that utilize the concept of working with parts to bring the multiplicity of our inner selves into alignment and balance. Dialogical Self Theory, developed by Hubert J.A. Hermans, examines the various positions of Self, parsing out the internalized voices of parental figures and noticing impulses within, which might manifest as an ambitious self or one who needs recognition (Hermans, 2012).

Chair work, based on Gestalt Therapy, creates a dialog between different parts by personifying an aspect of self or an inner voice and placing it in another chair. One client of mine was struggling with residual effects of a sexual assault several years earlier, which seemed to be impeding her as she prepared to marry. There was a part of her that felt like it was always on alert, generating self-blame, anxiety and panic attacks. She felt that this part was telling her that the assault had been her fault because she had been drinking, and therefore she was unworthy of her fiancé's love. How could she marry him if she was so "bad"?

I invited her to move to another chair and imagine that she was that wounded part. What was she saying to herself? She did this but quickly became uncomfortable. I asked if I could take on that persona and she said yes. I embodied that part and, using her words and tone, I told her everything was her fault and invited her to counter the argument of this disruptive part. She began talking back to that voice inside of her, embodied by me, saying she was not to blame. She told the part that she was in love, and she didn't need to be berated by the past. She told "me" to be quiet and that she was in charge. As her statements became stronger, I sank down, becoming smaller and eventually slipped behind the chair, effectively causing the "part" to disappear. As we processed this afterwards, my client felt relieved and released.

Another client, a former dancer, said her Inner Child longed to dance. The death of her father was complicated since he had abandoned his first family in favor of his second one. She felt this had caused her childlike part to become small and still so as not to attract attention amid family turmoil. We moved together with our eyes closed and she allowed that part of her to enter her body and dance freely. When we were finished, she was laughing and found this spontaneous dance enjoyable and freeing.

The Whole Self

What does it mean to feel whole? Abraham Maslow proposed that when the majority of our basic needs are met and we feel secure, loved and connected, we have the ability to become "self-actualized" (Bernstein *et al.*, 2003). To me, this means we can integrate all aspects of who we are and step into our Wise Self, integrating all aspects of our personal qualities, what and who we engage with and live from our Best Self.

Richard Schwartz (2022) describes it as follows:

[W]e suddenly encounter a feeling of inner plenitude and open heartedness to the world that wasn't there the moment before. The incessant nasty chatter inside our heads ceases, we have a sense of calm spaciousness, as if our minds and hearts and souls had expanded and brightened. Sometimes, these evanescent experiences come in a bright glow of peaceful certainty that

THE RINGS OF IDENTITY

everything in the universe is truly okay, and that includes us—you and me individually—in all our poor struggling, imperfect humanity. At other times, we may experience a wave of joyful connection with others that washes away irritation, distrust, and boredom. We feel that, for once, we truly are ourselves, our real selves, free of the inner cacophony that usually assaults us.

The Whole Self, or the Larger Self as Schwartz calls it, is the Leader. When we achieve that state of completeness, of luminosity and connection, we can allow the inner parts to stop being so cacophonous. By discovering the different ways in which we express our Self and by allowing our little selves to have a voice, we are able to truly step into the wholeness of who we are.

Internal Family Systems (IFS) Theory names these parts inside, with descriptors of their purpose for being. Schwartz explains these parts, saying that none of them are inherently bad even if they prevent us from engaging in fulfilling activities or in trying something new. The Self, the innate personality and the internal parts make up a system with subpersonalities that have thoughts, feelings and reactions. These parts are all trying to keep us safe, organized and happy. IFS Theory says we have Managers who keep us organized and strive for efficiency. Firefighter parts respond with alarms or even *with alarm* when we might be in danger or about to do something risky. Exiles are parts that have split off due to traumatic experiences, neglect or dissociation.

These parts can be recognized and their origins understood, but they are not separate from who we are. We are a jumble of all of our experiences, our shifting philosophies as we grew and responded to people and events throughout our life. We can describe who we are by naming what we do. When I was a dancer and would define myself as such, was I not also other aspects? I have written in journals for most of my life, yet I did not define myself as a writer until I finally decided to publish a book. When I ran a catering business, was I only a chef? I was also a mother, a sister, wife, friend. While part of me is involved in what I do, that is not the only definition of who I am.

In *The Creative Toolkit for Working with Grief and Bereavement*, I have a simple wheel comprised of two circles with spokes dividing them into sections (Coenen, 2020). I invite clients to reflect on the question "Who am I?" and to jot down whatever comes to mind in answer. This becomes a tool for discussing how they see themselves, how they present themselves to others, which invariably leads to an opening to who they might want to be in the

187

future. This is also a good way to begin to engage with aspects of our selves that seem to be younger or personifications of different aspects or "voices" that seem to exist within us.

We also can define ourselves by our qualities, by the type of person we believe we are. One client defined himself as thoughtful, careful, determined and helpful. He also defined himself as absentminded, cynical, anxious and stubborn. While some of these qualities might seem contradictory, they reflect the fact that we are not static and can hold opposite traits or characteristics within us. I believe that when we operate out of our Wise Self most of the time, we become the Leader of our multiplicity.

Noticing the internal messages we live with, reinforce and hold on to enables us to begin to step back and observe them. Is this message or way of reacting to others something that was laid on us by someone else? Where did this emotion or idea originate from? What or who is it connected to?

It can be effective to imagine that you are taking this message out of your mind or the emotion out of your body and placing it in the palm of your hand, held at some distance from yourself. I imagine placing my anger in my palm, acknowledging it by saying, "Hello, anger. Why are you here? What do you want me to know?" This small action enables me to have some distance from that emotion which is impeding my ability to think rationally and to respond rather than react with a sense of curiosity. "Oh, this is interesting. I wonder what I can learn from this?" is a different stance from simply becoming enraged and acting out.

In her book *The Wisdom of Anxiety*, Sheryl Paul (2019, p.132) offers the concept of an inner dining table where all the parts of ourselves are seated. Imagine that the younger parts, the wounded parts, the striving parts and the wise part are all there. They all have a reason for showing up to the dinner and they all have something important (at least to them) to say. When I begin to populate this metaphor, I notice that there often is one part clamoring to be heard—in fact, it may even have climbed up on to the tabletop. Look, she's jumping up and down and yelling. She thinks no one is listening and she is oblivious to the fact that she is not allowing anyone else to speak, let alone giving them time to turn their attention to her.

Because of my earlier work with Elizabeth in Talking Staff Circles, I like to conceptualize an internal Wisdom Circle. I imagine all my parts sitting around a small fire. Flickering light emanates off the fire as we gather around. I, the wise and grown-up part, remind everyone that each will have a chance to speak. We will take turns by passing on object, perhaps a shiny black stone. Each part can only speak while holding this stone and all the other members of the Wisdom Circle must listen with deep attention and compassion. I remind my Inner Voices that we will all listen with the ears of our hearts to each other speaking.

The Rings of Identity

Inviting a grieving client to focus on who they are after loss requires sensitivity. It is important to discern whether the client is ready for this kind of self-discovery, which could be developed over several sessions. Leave lots of room for reflection and for insight to arise within that reflection. There are no right answers to the question of "Who am I?" and contradictions or dissonances will arise. These can then be noticed and an inquiry into how these different aspects might come to the assistance of the whole can often be useful. Avoid judgment; invite your client to approach the discovery of their inner parts and inner inhabitants with curiosity.

This exercise will take several sessions with a client and can also be extended to private work between sessions. You might take a full session for the Outer Identity Ring and use the next session for processing, then the next session to consider the Relational Identity Ring.

This exercise is appropriate for clients who are able to conceptualize their Inner Parts and Voices and probably will not work in depth with children, although some of the ideas can be used with children if they mention a part of themselves or use a metaphor that evokes parts inside.

For the purposes of this exercise, three rings will be created. The fourth ring is the entire sphere, representing the Whole person.

Creating the Rings of Identity

Just as the Wheel of Identity (Coenen, 2020) invites a client to ask themselves "Who Am I?" and write their answers within the Wheel, the Rings of Identity takes the exploration of identity after loss to a deeper place. We will create three concentric circles, representing three aspects of identity, and then view the entire response as the Whole of who we are at this moment in time.

This creative exercise can be done with clients over a period of time. Some of the work can take place within a session and/or can be accomplished in reflective work between sessions. It would be wise to take your time as the client explores their realms of identity so that you can provide support, encouragement and grounding. Encourage journaling or another mode of reflection throughout the process. Allow time for the client to speak about how they view their identity, particularly the Inner Parts. You might use dialog techniques such as chair work or crossing a line between two parts so that the client's parts have the opportunity to say what they need to say.

You will need the following:

- A large piece of paper to trace a circle on or a large cardboard round. The circle should be at least 12 inches in diameter—the larger the better.
- Colored paper—construction paper or card stock. Have at least three colors.
- Pens and pencils, markers, colored pencils or pastels or any other media you like if you want to decorate your rings when complete.
- A notebook or some paper for reflection, either for writing or drawing.
- A glue stick or other adhesive.
- Tracing paper to trace the petal template, or you can draw your own shape to use. Note there are two sizes of petals. Feel free to use them both or choose the size that feels right for your circle.

Creating the Circles of Identity

1. Trace a circle on the paper if you are not using a cardboard round.
2. Choose at least three colors and trace the petal or your own preferred shape. Then cut out the petals you want to use. Cut out 6–12 petals in each color. Use one color for the outer ring, another for the next ring and a third color for the inner ring. If you wish, you can use multiple colors.
3. Consider each Ring of Identity. Take your time but don't overthink. Using a journal or piece of paper, write down what arises in each of the three realms. Write each aspect or quality on a petal.
4. Arrange the petals on the circle, beginning with the outermost ring. Glue the petals onto the large circle. This can be done after each ring is investigated. The petals of the next ring can overlap the previous ring or not.
5. You might enjoy decorating any bare areas on the page or in between

the petals if you wish. You are also free to name your parts and add other aspects or qualities that might appear while reflecting on the rings.

TEMPLATE FOR RINGS OF IDENTITY

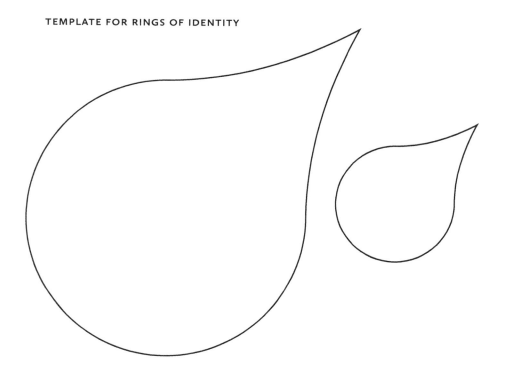

The First Ring—the Outer Identity

This ring represents how we operate in the world and how we present ourselves. This includes what we do in the world, our jobs or careers, how we act and what qualities we embody when we are in the outer realm. What do we say when we introduce ourselves to someone else? How do we describe ourselves to others and to ourselves? Some people define themselves in the outer ring by their professions. Some might also define themselves by how they accomplish their work, saying they are diligent, focused, compassionate, detail oriented. Remember, there are no incorrect answers.

Ask the following questions:

- Who am I in the world?

- What do I do in the world that defines me?

The Second Ring—the Relational Identity

In this ring, we focus on who are we in relationship with and how we operate in the relationships. Some of the definitions might overlap with the Outer Identity—for example, in the outer ring I am a counselor, and in this ring, I relate to my clients with compassion and interest. In my Relational Identity, I might say I am a mother, grandmother, sister, friend. I am still a widow, and I am also a wife. When I define *how* I relate, I could add that I am a good listener, I am organized, inquisitive, impatient, mindful and sometimes angry and sharp.

Ask:

- Who am I in relationship with and how does that define me?
- How am I in relationship? These could be qualities you bring to your relationships.

The Third Ring—My Inner Wisdom Circle

Who inhabits the innermost sanctum of your Self? Whether you see this as an Inner Dining Table or a Wisdom Circle, allow your imagination to call up these parts of you. You may find a much younger part of yourself or identify the cautious part or the one that is afraid of change. Invite them in and seat them.

If it feels right, name the parts that inhabit the innermost Ring of Identity. This helps to personify them as "others" in order to allow them to speak. This also generates curiosity into who they are and where they came from. One client identified Little Miss Perfect, who must always please everyone and do things properly. Another part, Big Girl Panties, berates her if she feels sad, telling her she should just move on. Concrete Being tries hard to keep her safe from the traumas she has experienced and the people who perpetrated them, but Concrete Being also prevents her from experiencing happiness or from taking chances. By identifying and engaging with these various parts, the client had a chance to dialog with them from her Wise position, lessening their ability to truly engage with her life now.

In my own Wisdom Circle, I find an Angry Teen, a Twirling Child, a part that always wants to know "WHY," whom I have named "Whynona." I have invited my Widow part and my Healer part to have a seat around the imaginary fire. The Wise Woman is in the Wisdom Circle, and I want her to be the timekeeper and guide for the others.

Once the inner Wisdom Circle has been populated, explore each "person." What does this part of yourself look like? What are they wearing? How does their body sit or move? How old are they? Enter into a dialog with that part and ask for its contributing message. Listen compassionately, as you would with a friend in pain. Speak back to it, letting it know that you have heard its message. If you disagree or are in a different place in your life now, let that part know this. Let your most wounded and underdeveloped parts know that you have grown.

Conversing with inner parts can help reduce their interfering activation and create a path towards their integration.

Ask:

- Who are the different parts of me that speak up the most or call for attention?
- How old are they?
- What name should I give each part?

The Fourth Ring or the Whole Multiplicity of Self

The Fourth Ring of Identity is the entire circle. Once you have engaged with three levels of identity, you can view the Whole You. Notice what has been written and what feels congruent. Notice disparities, dissonances and contradictions. How can you bring these into balance? Are there other parts that are hiding and have not revealed themselves? How will you integrate all the parts of your Self, once you have listened with the ears of your heart to these other voices?

We can integrate the multiple aspects of our selves and bring our parts into alignment. We can develop a sense of wholeness as we engage in this process. Yet it is important to remember that we will fluctuate and dip. A wounded part may be activated and scream for attention at inopportune moments. Our Inner Critic may step in front of us just before we are about to give a presentation at work or try something new. If we are mindful of the internal members of our own Wisdom Circle, we will develop skills for coping with this "intrusion." Our multiplicity shows up for a reason. It is up to our Wise Self to decide to be curious about this, when to listen and when to kindly ask that part to sit down. Thank it first for showing up!

You can journal your response to Rings of Identity once it is complete. The journal does not have to be a narrative; it can be a word or two that resonates with each realm. It could be a poem. It could be a drawing in color, a visualization of your integrated Whole Self.

References

Arrien, A. (2008). The Soul's Fire: Bring Meaning, Magic and Majesty into the World. In K. Steinnes (ed.) *Women of Wisdom: Empowering the Dreams and Spirit of Women*. Seattle, WA: Wise Woman Publishing.

Bernstein, D.A., Penner, L.A., Clarke-Stewart, A., & Roy, E.J. (2003). *Psychology*. Boston, MA: Houghton Mifflin.

Coenen, C. (2018). *Shattered by Grief: Picking up the Pieces to Become WHOLE Again*. London and Philadelphia, PA: Jessica Kingsley Publishers.

Coenen, C. (2020). *The Creative Toolkit for Working with Grief and Bereavement: A Practitioner's Guide*. London and Philadelphia, PA: Jessica Kingsley Publishers.

Cogburn, E. (1984). Warriors of the beauty way: Realizing the power of human potential by creating in beauty. An interview with Elizabeth Cogburn by Ross Chapin. *Art and Ceremony in Sustainable Culture*, Spring. www.context.org/iclib/ic05/cogburn

Hermans, H.J. (2012). *Between Dreaming and Recognition Seeking: The Emergence of Dialogical Self Theory*. Lanham, MD: University Press of America.

Koff-Chapin, D. (1983). Living with Ceremonial and Finding Depth. *In Context: Being a Planetary Villager*, December. www.context.org/iclib/ic01/chapin

Parkes, C.P. (2010). *Bereavement: Studies of Grief in Adult Life*. London: Penguin.

Paul, S. (2019). *The Wisdom of Anxiety: How Worry and Intrusive Thoughts Are Gifts to Help You Heal*. Boulder, CO: Sounds True.

Schwartz, R. (2021). *Investigating Internal Family Systems*. Rhinebeck, NY: Omega Institute.

Schwartz, R. (2022, July 22). The Larger Self. IFS Institute. https://ifs-institute.com/resources/articles/larger-self

CHAPTER 14

Out of Grief Comes Art

Elizabeth Coplan

I am not an academic with advanced degrees or a researcher in the clinical sense. What I am is an observer of life.

Eight years ago, I experienced three deaths in one year. Although I was willing to share my stories of those losses, no one wanted to hear them. It was as if death was contagious. So I channeled my grief into writing a play. My early love of theatre allowed me to pivot easily to playwriting. I was drafting *Over My Dead Body* when I found myself stuck on how to work through a particular scene.

To overcome this block, I wrote a separate epilogue between the two sisters in the play, a scene I never meant to include in the original script. I showed this ten-minute script to some theatre friends who encouraged me to submit it to various short play festivals. The show won many of the festivals all across the U.S. and enjoyed a six-week run at the Group Rep Theater in North Hollywood.

It shocked me when I realized that each time I attended a performance and the audience learned I was the playwright, they gathered to talk to me. They wanted to share their own stories of grief and loss. These stories ranged from funny to tragic, often both. Occasionally, the loss was recent. Other times, it happened years ago—the grief still lodged in their throats as they spoke of their loved ones and the circumstances around the deaths.

This realization was both humbling and inspiring. My play held healing power not merely in the dialogue but in its ability to create a visceral response within those watching the production.

If my story could bring this much shared experience over death and grief, think what the addition of other people's stories could provide audiences. So I contacted several playwrights, and we assembled an evening of short plays depicting various scenarios of dying, death, and/or grief, which launched Grief Dialogues.

In 2020, Honoring Choices PNW, a Washington State nonprofit, commissioned me to write a stage play about end-of-life planning. I wrote the play *Honoring Choices* based on the story of my own father's terminal diagnosis. We performed the show live during their February 2020 conference and on Zoom throughout 2021. Again, audience members shared their stories of loved ones and their end-of-life trials and regrets. The play clearly resonated, and more people shared their stories about advanced care planning. The demand for the play sparked interest in creating a film, and in 2022, I learned the art of screenwriting to create the film version.

My artistic/creative focus is always theatre and now film. But theatre is not the only art form that helps us understand our emotions. Recent studies demonstrate the intrinsic benefits in all types of art including visual media, music, and movement. A World Health Organization (WHO) report (Fancourt & Finn, 2019) synthesizes the global evidence on the role of the arts in improving health and wellbeing, with a specific focus on the WHO European Region. Results from more than 3000 studies identified a major role for the arts in the prevention of ill health, promotion of health, and management and treatment of illness across the lifespan. The reviewed evidence included study designs such as uncontrolled pilot studies, case studies, small-scale cross-sectional surveys, nationally representative longitudinal cohort studies, community-wide ethnographies, and randomized controlled trials from diverse disciplines. The beneficial impact of the arts could be furthered through acknowledging and acting on the growing evidence base; promoting arts engagement at the individual, local, and national levels; and supporting cross-sectoral collaboration. These studies show how the arts can reduce stress, prevent or slow the progression of a range of medical conditions including mental illness, and effectively treat depression and anxiety.

What is art? Its interpretation varies throughout history and across cultures. I describe art as an activity that involves a creative process—one that demonstrates emotional power and/or conceptual ideas. Engagement in any creative process bridges our body, mind, and spirit, building into an art form. Creating art out of our anguish and loss is profoundly cathartic and reinforces our resilience whether we share our creation or not. Many artists have used their personal sorrow and adverse experiences to create some of their greatest work.

I have interviewed different artists to represent how grief became art. Below are edited versions of their responses.

Each grief story (Remembering) is different. The why and how each artist makes their art is also diverse. Similarly, what the art means to each artist resonates differently (Reflections).

None of the artists are household names, but all are professionals in every sense of the word. All of them stress the vital importance of art in helping them process grief, and each artist offered their suggestions (Recommendations) for the casual artist, the never-before-artist, and the returning artist.

Grief is an incredibly intense, all-consuming feeling, and feeling drives art. Art in turn gives the invisible, hard to articulate inner experience a tangible physical presence. In truth, out of grief comes art.

Artist: Caito Stewart
Art: Mixed Media Art

REMEMBERING—CAITO'S GRIEF STORY

When I was 13, my younger brother died in an accident on a playdate with a friend. He was only nine years old. He had fallen into a ravine, only a ten-minute walk away from our house. A month earlier, during Hurricane Floyd, a car had been swept into this ravine that feeds into the Hudson River. The boys had heard about this car and decided to go looking for it. Andrew fell about 80 feet. He hit his head and we couldn't save him.

My family were Christian Scientists and did not believe in going to doctors or using medicine to heal anything. When my brother was airlifted to the hospital, my mother had a lot of guilt since in her mind she should not have allowed him to be taken to the hospital in the first place. She felt that was the reason he had died.

Art is what helped me regulate my emotions. In Christian Science, you are not supposed to have negative emotions or acknowledge the material body, death, sadness, grief, or anger. I did not have anybody to talk to about my brother. That all went into my art and some of it was pretty dark.

It was a very scary and traumatic time for all of us. We all felt the anger and anxiety. I fled to Japan after college and made a new life for myself. In Japan, I became an educator and an artist.

When my mom died suddenly in 2017, I didn't know that she had been struggling with her health. I knew she had a heart attack five years earlier, but my parents had minimized the severity of it and made it sound as if she had healed it. "She's good," they would tell me. "Look at her. She's lost all this weight. She's good. Don't worry. You don't need to come home."

I had lived ten years in Tokyo when my mother suddenly died. I felt completely paralyzed. Everything changed in that moment. I thought I was going to live in Japan forever. I loved my job, but suddenly, I couldn't work. I couldn't do anything. My leg stopped working—literally. When I went home for the memorial service and then returned to Japan, my leg was swollen and I wasn't able to work for a month. I was on crutches. I went to many doctors to understand why my leg would not move.

The only thing I could do was paint. Thinking, processing, and mourning. Painting was the only thing I cared about. I knew I had to quit my job and leave. I packed up my whole life, said goodbye to everything I loved, and started over again, back in a country where I wasn't sure I could fit in anymore.

I knew I had to face the past. I had to face my brother's death, the [continuing] family conflict and how my mother intentionally kept everything from us because it would "hinder her healing if we knew about it and had any fear around it."

I lived with my dad briefly in our childhood home, where my younger brother's ashes are scattered under the maple tree in the front yard. It was hard to overcome all the memories. I found it difficult to live there.

My brother wrote a screenplay inspired by our family history, so I know that was something creative that helped him process our trauma.

In 2018, I moved to Brooklyn and received my MFA in sculpture at Pratt in the middle of the pandemic in 2020. Our thesis shows were canceled and all classes moved online. We lost access to our studios for the entire last semester and it was devastating. More grief.

Painting was what got me through the grief the first time around and through all the conflict since, that embroiled our family for years.

REFLECTIONS

Why do you make your art?
I don't think I could stay sane if I didn't make my art. I also make music. I'm in a band. I write the vocals and the lyrics. I tap into a lot of different things, but without all these outlets, I think that I would explode.

How do you make it?

My art helps me understand my grief and helps me process and heal. A lot of thinking and writing goes into making the artwork, too. I don't just paint or make something. It is very conceptual for me. I need to feel an experience. How can I conceptually convey an idea?

I often write out memories, lists of things, and think about visual imagery or objects, especially everyday objects that have meaning to me, but may also have different associations or meanings to other people. I brainstorm it until I have an image that hits me.

I mainly brainstorm by myself, but I also talk about it with friends or artist friends or my partner. They are my sounding boards. We discuss concepts about the body and mental health. I also like to talk about nature and what things in nature symbolize. I think about the devastation of fire and how certain things grow right afterwards, pioneer species like fungi and mushrooms.

I have lots of connections to food. One piece I am working on now is a giant bag of Pop Secret microwaveable popcorn. I'm making the bag out of paper and then painting the design.

The bag is about four by six feet. It will sit on the floor or hang from the ceiling. I am also making these popcorn kernels out of ceramic clay. I take actual kernels of popcorn and I observe them and I make each one at a time. Each sculpture of a kernel is at least three inches in diameter.

I observe the textures and little nooks and crannies. I make each kernel individually in different textures and shapes. Some are un-popped, still encased in a shiny shell. Some are fluffy and not shiny, maybe with a bit of butter on it. There's something cathartic about looking at these things that have such beauty in them. Observing these organic shapes is meditative for me. It takes me out of everything I am dealing with and brings me to the present moment. I appreciate looking at something in a new way that I never have before.

Normally, I just eat popcorn and don't pay attention to how they look. When I look at the kernels, they are actually quite beautiful. There are so many associations surrounding food that are personal to me. I spent time with my mother connecting through food because that was the one comfort she allowed herself. I have wonderful memories of the two of us sitting on the couch with a bowl of Pop Secret, watching movies.

At the same time, there are complications around it, too. I am mad at her for not teaching me to have a better diet, eat healthier, and take care of my body. She didn't take care of hers and it ultimately led to her death.

This popcorn concept is double-edged. I enjoy these different levels of meanings. I like that each kernel can have a different meaning. If one is un-popped, it means it has "unused potential." If it's half popped, it's not quite there, and if it's fully popped, it has realized its potential. If it's not there, it means it was consumed. There is an aspect of impermanence in popcorn.

There's an uncertainty with clay that I enjoy. In my art I spend a lot of time trying to contain things and encapsulate and preserve and stop the decay or the loss. There's also something about the thrill, the not knowing and the hoping and the challenge that I like, too.

It could be a metaphor for parts of myself or my relationship with my mother and her life or life in general. I leave it up to interpretation for the viewers. But I enjoy playing with the ideas and the images, the challenge of trying to figure out how to make this thing.

From my art, I've developed resilience and perseverance because it's hard to be an artist in this world. You must have this fire in you, this need to keep doing it, to keep searching and trying to create. In the past, I've called my art many different things, but now I use the word "reliquary." To me it means a beautiful container.

RECOMMENDATIONS

I am also an art educator. Sometimes art is merely observing, an act of mindfulness. It's a muscle like any other skill; you have to practice and learn by doing. Start with a still life or grab a cool rock and some watercolors. Try to paint it—draw it. Keep it simple.

Art can be learning something new, like a language. When I was learning Japanese, every time I said a sentence that I'd never said before and expressed a new thought I had never expressed, I said: "Wow. I did that. I can do this. Let's keep going."

Artist: Steve Jensen
Art: Artist (Sculpture)
REMEMBERING—STEVE'S GRIEF STORY
Content warning: This story describes suicide.

My family is from Norway, fishermen and boat builders. Upon the death of both of my parents, I made a boat for their ashes, took it out to sea and sank it, something like a contemporary Viking funeral. I also made one for my former partner of 24 years and one for my best friend who died of AIDS two years later. It was the same month my father put a gun in his mouth and shot himself.

Two years and two days after my father's suicide, my mom fell apart. Emotionally, physically. I had to commit her three times to a mental institution. Actually, in America, you can't really commit your parent, so I had to convince her to commit herself, which really made it ten times more painful.

My former partner was a heavy drinker, and the day before he died, he asked me to make a boat for him. And he wanted to be buried with my mom and dad in the same place in the same manner.

REFLECTIONS

Why do you make your art?
The boat is the symbolic voyage or journey to the other side. I'm attempting to take something that is extremely painful and turn it into something beautiful. I hope the take-away of my work is that when something tragic, something painful, happens, turn your energy into something positive, something beautiful.

Right now, we live in an era where a million people died in the United States in 2020 (CDC, 2022). We need to take that energy and do something positive, acknowledge those deaths and do something positive with that energy.

I'm extremely dyslexic and I have been since early childhood. I always thought I was just stupid. Art allows me to express myself. Also, as a child I was extremely shy, and art allowed me to express myself and to get my thoughts out.

I also have trouble writing. Even turning on a computer is complicated for me. When I write on a computer, I can't even get close enough to the correct spelling of a word in order to spellcheck it. Art has been a way for me, my entire life, to express my feelings and to express myself.

I am currently focusing on the boats, embracing my heritage. Originally, my name was Finn Sen. My parents changed it to Steve in the 1960s when they were trying to assimilate into America.

How do you make it?

A friend dying in hospice gave me a drawing of a boat and said, "When I die, I want you to make a boat for my ashes and I want to be buried at sea." He died a week later, and I made the boat. I tried to make it as close to his drawing as possible.

My mom was so moved by this boat that she wanted a boat for my father's ashes when he died. The boat was the obvious choice since he was a fisherman and a boat builder. My mother asked me to make a boat for her ashes, which I took out to sea and sank.

My mom's memorial boat, which is probably the most sentimental, is covered with all her joy. It has a plaster cast of her face that I made in art school, 20 years earlier, which I covered with photocopies of her death certificate. I made a shroud out of a painting on silk from the 1950s. The boat had her driver's license, a family photo from her wallet, and her old-fashioned watch that required winding. It was still working when she died.

My friend's memorial boat contained some of his personal effects when he died—his comb, his toothbrush. The day we knew he would die, he looked terrible, and I had a hairdresser friend come and give him a haircut and a shave. I was cleaning up the hair off of the floor and put it in my pocket and incorporated that into his memorial boat. It spells out the word AIDS in his hair.

The ships are like ghost ships to me. The people in my life are physically gone, but they're always with me, and I ask for their help. My friend helps me with art. My dad helps me with working and sometimes physically making the art because he was a boat builder. My mom helps me with my emotions and my feelings. My former partner was very wealthy, and he helps me with money. I ask for help and they come help me.

Good art makes you feel something, think something. And if it doesn't, it is just wallpaper.

RECOMMENDATIONS

Express your thoughts, however you can and by whatever means you can. If it's drawing or painting, singing, dancing, whatever you can do. Turn these emotions into something beautiful. It doesn't have to be high quality.

Here's an example of how powerful creating art can be. I did a major public art piece at a boy's prison for the Washington State Arts Commission and was asked to be an artist in residence at the prison. I designed a program to make self-portrait masks and storyboards. I would give them the starting points and they'd find objects and make a mask of themselves. As we worked together, the students created their own original pieces, and I was honored to share their work in several museum shows.

Art will never bring anyone back, but it is a shield against silence and forgetting.

Any creative process gives us a break from cogitating, talking, and doing to simply be in the moment by taking part in our artistic practice. It can act as the thread between in our heads, hearts, and hands. Reflecting on the outcome of our creative process often enables us to tell our story and process our emotions outside the moments of loss and grief.

Artist: Kathryn Keats

Art: Performance Art (Songwriter, Playwright, Performer, Singer, and Composer)

REMEMBERING—KATHRYN'S GRIEF STORY

I landed in New York in my teens following the death of my older brother. I arrived in the city carrying an immense amount of grief. My brother and I had a big fight the day he died. He had begged me to take him to school so he wouldn't have to ride his motorcycle in the rain. I refused. On his way home, he was hit by a van in the rain. I stopped eating the next day. My mother stopped talking.

The only thing I ever wanted to do was sing. Six months after my brother's death, I talked my mother into driving me from Indiana to NYC so I could pursue my dream of performing on Broadway. I was cast in an off-Broadway show and fell in love with the music director. I was 18 years old, and he was much older than me. He quickly became my mentor and my lover, and I became his muse.

We were prolifically creative. We wrote music and shows, and our collaboration was one of the most rewarding creative experiences of my life. Unbeknownst to me, he had bipolar disorder and was schizophrenic. As his disease progressed, I tried to save him from the horrific pain he experienced. His health rapidly became the epicenter of my life, my sole reason for existing. The relationship became volatile. The voices that were haunting him had convinced him I was at the center of a conspiracy trying to control him. He said I needed to be dismembered and hung from the trees. He had several personalities, all extremely abusive. Yet I loved him. And that meant I had to save him.

He held me in our apartment for 54 days. My sister rescued me. My captor was arrested, and a jury trial followed. I changed my identity in order to disappear. It was the only thing that could keep me safe. I left my career, my friendships, and life as I had known it. Ultimately, my safety was entirely up to me. The post-traumatic stress I experienced was paralyzing. I was underground for 20 years. When I found out he had passed, I emerged and finally sang again. I was free.

Or so I had hoped. Despite his death, the work that lay ahead was monumental. Through self-reflection, therapy, and art, a thread between my brother's accident and my lover's death became visible. The shame and guilt I felt at the loss of my brother catalyzed my obsessive need to save my lover. I had a mistaken sense of responsibility. It was a disservice to us both.

I wrote and recorded an album called *After the Silence* and then began working on my solo beat musical, *The Hummingbird*, which details the story of my experience with my music-partner lover. It took ten years to complete. It began in residency at Berkeley Repertory. I play 15 characters in the show, which has proved paramount in the emotional and psychological unraveling of my story. *The Hummingbird* won Best Solo Musical at the 2021 International Marshstream Festival.

REFLECTIONS

Why do you make your art?

Nerve endings are longer than my appendages, and making art helps me maintain a certain amount of equilibrium. If I don't create, I feel like I don't exist. Creating art allows me to break rules. And I'm a big rule breaker. I'm drawn to creative works that don't mind their manners. I like messy work.

How do you make it?

I make art by surrendering. Whether it's songs, poetry, plays, or music, I enjoy an almost trance-like state and art comes through. At the same time, years of study and discipline allow me the gift of focus.

I started very young. In fact, I started making art as a performer when

I was five. I loved it. I was a singer and a performer, and I started studying to be an artist at five. When I was in my late teens, I started writing music and songs and writing shows.

My voice was not as great as it could have been when my first album, *After the Silence*, came out, but the band was incredible. And then I wrote a book, or at least I started to write a book.

I turned the book into a multi-person show. While I was in residency at Berkeley Repertory Ground Floor, I decided to turn this piece into a solo show. But I'd been in hiding so long that I really didn't know how to be out in the world. Trying to do it at Berkeley Rep with a group was really difficult for me because I was so used to being isolated.

Fortunately for me, I started working with David Ford on my solo show. I told the story of what happened in the music, in the song. It's a beat musical with lyric and book, which is written in almost a beat poetry form because that's how I happen to write. It is how I naturally write.

I am drawn to rap as a musician, and I am drawn to slam poetry and I am drawn to really discombobulated types of writing.

RECOMMENDATIONS

When it comes to using art as a way to work through grief and pain, I suggest you try anything you can do, whether it's writing, drawing—it can be hammering a stick into the ground. Even if you don't think it's art, it probably is art. If you don't think you can sing and you want to sing, then don't let anyone stop you.

If you do nothing else, just show up! Get out. Share with people.

Artist: Laurel Marlantes
Art: Writing

REMEMBERING—LAUREL'S GRIEF STORY

My grief was like a hundred-pound invisible weight I dragged around, hoping it would make me invisible, too. I had given birth to a stillborn child. I was grieving a life no one else had known, cared about, or connected with. How could I even begin to share or explain the pain in my heart? Was I even allowed to be this destroyed, so completely debilitated by grief, over a life that technically never lived? I judged my grief. To further complicate things, my stillbirth was the result of a late-term abortion due to medical complications affecting the viability of the baby's life. It was a choice my husband and I made together, from the most profound love we had ever encountered, yet culture's message was clear on this one: that part of your story is something you keep silent. For years, we did—the silence compounding the weight my broken heart carried.

Handing my son's little body over for the last time was the most painful moment of my life, as were the weeks that followed as my body recovered from labor and continued to make milk for a baby that wasn't there. His birth, though, is my life's most treasured and holy moment. I experienced birth and death simultaneously, my soul and heart stretching wider than I ever knew I could.

REFLECTIONS

Why do you make your art?

After my stillbirth, there was a part of me that always just felt broken and alone. Writing my story helped me pull these fragmented parts of myself back together. Sharing it is my way of trying to help both myself and others feel not so alone. Stories have a unique ability to heal. They do not tell you how to act, feel, or behave—they take you on a journey, one that allows a listener or reader to extract their own truths, teachings, and medicine from. Universal truths are revealed through story in a way that is soft and relatable, reminding us how connected we are, nourishing our sense of belonging.

How do you make it?

What I do is designate time for the task. Some days the writing flows more than others, and I've learned to accept that and realize I don't have control over which days those are, only over whether or not I show up. I know that nothing will happen if I don't.

Showing up for me is first and foremost. Second, especially if I'm struggling with a particular part, I set a timer for ten minutes and sit in silence and ground myself. Writing, especially getting that first draft down, takes bravery, and I'm always braver after giving myself a moment to root and connect. Memoir writing is like going on a hunt for the deepest truth in your life experience and then searching for words to communicate that truth. It requires emotional vulnerability and strength. You might not always like what you find. But I've learned if I keep going, tethering myself to a place of love and what it is my soul really wants to say, the hunt to find those honest words becomes easier.

Writing my story allowed me first to find my truth and now to stand comfortably in it. It's helped me emerge out of a dark night of the soul into a sense of groundedness I never thought possible. It's given me the unforeseen gift of becoming my own witness. Through the writing process, I came to see my story through a slightly detached, zoomed-out lens and, in doing so, see how worthy of love and voice it was. Even if no one ever reads the book, knowing I found the words to my truth and hearing my own voice speak that truth has been profoundly healing—worth every minute and agonizing moment the writing held.

RECOMMENDATIONS

Know that doing anything might feel impossible, and that's OK. Small steps are big wins. If possible, clear a space for yourself and designate it as a place you can go when you don't know what to do with yourself. A place, as my mother once told me, you can "get out of your head, out of your heart, and into your hands." Have a candle there, one you can light for yourself or in honor of the loved one you've lost, and then pick up the pen, paints, or knitting needles, whatever simple creative task feels approachable, and let the medium's rhythm take over.

Artist: Robert A. Neimeyer
Art: Poetry

REMEMBERING—ROBERT'S GRIEF STORY

Like most people, I have known a litany of losses in my time—of people, places, projects, possessions, and even professions that once anchored the core meanings of my life. These have been quite variegated, ranging from the death of my paternal grandmother in our home when I was eight, through the suicide of my father when I was 11, to the death of my mother from COPD (chronic obstructive pulmonary disease) when I was in full adulthood, and the parent of young children. And, of course, a host of non-death losses—among the most anguishing of them the demise of hoped-for life partnerships—have prompted their own forms of desolation and called for deep emotional processing. My art (if it can be dignified with that term) has most commonly arisen in the wake of these turbulent transitions, as I strive to discern the lessons of loss, so to speak.

REFLECTIONS

Why do you make your art?

I usually feel drawn to the notebook or sketchbook against my will, in a sense, knowing that I'll be spending some uncomfortable minutes or hours doing something that involves more perspiration than inspiration.

I believe that grief has a need to be witnessed—if only by the griever. Some people, myself included, are heartened and held by the empathic witnessing of another.

Art created during my grief often brings out the messy human-ness—the anger, the unresolved wounds. And therapeutic art, at least, commonly arises from that messiness, that cauldron of emotion and undigested experience. Art transmutes that, potentially, into something resonant, true, and informative—even if painful. There's beauty in that—but it is the beauty one sees in an old, wizened, care-worn but knowing visage, rather than the Botoxed beauty of the Hollywood starlet. It's the studied gaze or sudden glance that reveals the latent structure of things, or the attuned ear that filters the noise to hear the true signal.

Art begins where we are, not where we want to be. Holding that in the now—in spoken word poetry, free verse, a quick sketch, a self-portrait, a complex collage—lets us come into fuller contact with ourselves, making sense of the experience and of ourselves in its presence. Once produced, the artwork then stands outside us, and invites a dialogue with what we do not yet know or understand. Most commonly, there is a message in it for our lives, and sometimes for the lives of others, if we are brave enough to look or listen for it. Perhaps the following poem hints at the inherent messiness of this process.

Old Shoes

I'm wearing old shoes and will for a while yet
the grief still holding close.

Sometimes when the longing for a single living thing
overcomes me like a sudden hunger I shuffle from the black mirror
to the long grass, painted in dew

and jerk the mower into a sputtering roar as I walk the tight lines
feet slipping in the mud just to smell the cut grass

remove it in clots from the black bag and hold it,
just a moment more like memories

before releasing it to compost.

How do you make it?

Genuine art is not simply technical proficiency. It issues from a place of mystery rather than mastery, from the not-yet-fully sensed, the partly non-conscious, the intuitive impulse, or the unfathomed need, more than from conscious design.

Sometimes I might find myself moved or caught up in a moment of encounter with the natural or human world, or an image will arise unbidden to capture it and give rein to the musings that follow from the simple act of perception. Occasionally, it is a simple *cri de coeur*, which conveys more commonly in first-person description what I do rather than what I feel, literally. It hints at internal states revealed in actions rather than a straightforward description of emotions. Sometimes I marinate in a metaphor that captures a mood, a stance, or a relationship better than literal language can, or at least more memorably.

But more commonly, I pick up the pen, pencil, or paintbrush when something is welling up within me that demands recognition, expression, validation, and sometimes working through. Grief is among the strongest of those calls. Rarely do my poems, sketches, paintings, or collages console or paper over the fissures in my heart in such moments; if anything, they accentuate them, name them, and claim them as my reality in that lived instant. But their meaning evolves as I do, and I commonly see different significance in them looking back than I did at the time I gave them voice or image.

RECOMMENDATIONS

1. Be the compassionate audience you seek.
2. Tell the truth of your life and your loss. And then let it change.
3. Pre-think nothing. Let the blank page call to the silent voices within you.
4. Write where it hurts. Find the place of most genuine feeling that lives in your body, and let it find words.

5. Be inclusive. When one inner voice finds expression on the page and falls silent, ask, "Who else is in there who has a response to this?" Trust that the most basic words of wisdom, perspective, and direction you need may be your own.

Artist: Robert Pardi
Art: Writing and Leadership Training
REMEMBERING—ROBERT'S GRIEF STORY

I chose a job on Wall Street out of anger to get away from my dad. For me, money was going to save me. Desiree and I fell in love, and her love helped me start to peel away, to sculpt my life into something that wasn't about my anger. When she became ill, I became introspective. I had to make the best of our lives.

It was living with her illness and subsequent death that the art form took over. I gave up the Wall Street job to be with her, to provide the best for her, and make a different life for specifically her. This is when the art really started.

REFLECTIONS

Why do you make your art?

Art is as simple as finding beauty in something. We're all artists, because if we are conscious and intentional about our lives and the way we build them, we are building a mosaic. We are painting a picture. I think art allows us to express our uniqueness and individuality.

I believe that beauty is in imperfection. I don't think art is perfect. Art evokes emotion. Perfection cannot evoke emotion.

I live in Italy and see ancient mosaics. Each stone was cut by hand, imperfect. These imperfections create the depth and uniqueness, making the mosaics appealing and attractive. My art and working with people help me understand their uniqueness.

How do you make it?

I'm a sculptor. That means that I chip away things that don't resonate with me. I strip away to get to what I see in the marble, like Michelangelo. He saw David within the marble.

My art is being intentional, and it's through being conscious that I understand awareness. I know who I am and what my uniqueness is, how to express that, what's satisfying to me. It's expressing something to the world. I'm using the tools of conscious living. I am intentional about how I live my life. I'm expressing my own light. People are attracted to the light, and they will come closer. The people who need sunglasses are going to go away.

When you are more intentional, you are more conscious, you're more aware, and you begin to realize, how can I be creative today?

Nobody can ever have life balance, but you can have harmony, like a beautiful, harmonious song, a symphony. What makes it harmonious is space, silence, and letting go of the last key, the last string. You need silence and the space between the notes.

My life sometimes hurts. Desiree passing away was a sucker punch.

Be the artist of your life. For me, my leadership work, life coaching, speaking, writing books are all expressions of who I am, of a passion inside of me. I write books as much for myself as I do for others. And because one of my core values is connection, my books are going to connect with people in an authentic way. I think a lot about what it means to be an artist. I do believe that artists see possibility and opportunities in things that other people don't see.

Art requires vulnerability. Grief was a call to action. I became the artist and accepted vulnerability because it all ends one day anyway. So why not show up as our authentic self and craft the life we want to live? Grief is like Kintsugi—it is letting go of something and making something even more beautiful, more unique out of it.

Vulnerability triggers emotions. I created as an acronym for GRIEF: G—guilt. R—rumination. I—impermanence. E—expectations. F—fear.

To walk through that is vulnerability. As I walk through the valley of the shadow of death, it is not death. It's vulnerability. Because everything you knew is no longer there. And that's where you become the artist.

RECOMMENDATIONS

I recommend constructive daydreaming. Imagination is the foundation of art. Positive constructive daydreaming opens us to experience life, to explore ideas, feelings. It improves problem solving, expands creativity, decreases stress, and enhances one's ability to reach goals. It is a tool that allowed me to care for Desiree and move forward with her loss. I reimagined my life living in Italy after my wife passed away. I imagined using my experience to help people. That allowed me to start to fill a big hole in my life with little dreams, little possibilities. We can't refill and will never refill a big loss or life change; it becomes part of us. The trap we fall into is wanting to "recover." Instead, I suggest starting to constructively daydream and place little nuggets of joy and wonder in that big space and starting to craft a new part of your mosaic, piece by piece.

Artist: Katie Pettit
Art: Dance
REMEMBERING—KATIE'S GRIEF STORY

Theatre, dance, and movement are how I tell stories. I love performing, but I am more interested in curating, creating, and being a part of how, why, and what's happening. I was directing and choreographing other people's work when I realized that their work did not have any real purpose beyond entertainment. I wanted my art to mean something more, bigger than my own interests. Working on Broadway was very eye-opening for me. It definitely revealed a lot of disparities. There was no Black or Brown representation or anyone else besides Caucasian people there.

This was devastating to my creative spirit. I realized that Broadway was not my pathway. It wasn't accessible, inclusive, or representative of how I wanted to create. I wanted to create work for marginalized folks who deserve a platform to be centered and celebrated. I founded my company, Katharine Pettit Creative—KPC, which equally stands for "Keeping People Connected." We use dance as our universal language.

Changing minds by opening hearts through movement is really what we are all about. I began to create a new dance musical, *I Could Never Love Anyone...* It is part of a quote from *Little Women*: "I could never love anyone as I love my sisters." My sisters and I would often say this phrase to each other.

Initially, we performed at theaters and festivals, but it wasn't what I wanted because at the end of the day, I wanted the art to speak to more people going through these lived experiences. People would come up to talk with me after the performances: "Oh my gosh. You know, I had my brother, a father, and I'm dealing with that."

Touring through the school systems make a massive impact on the young people. We continue to create and present what we now call our "Pathway to Wellness through Movement."

I lead everyone through emotionally guided movement exercises. You don't have to be a dancer or performer of any kind. We talk through different emotions like childhood joy, love, anger. And we ask people to think about someone they hadn't seen in a really long time. How would they react if that person came through the door? What sounds would you make and what might your body do?

We talk about a childhood memory where they feel safe and taken care of. We move through grief. The very first piece of *I Could Never Love Anyone...* is aptly called "There Will Be Tears."

Movement is an accessible entry point to reach the trauma, the emotions, and grief, and helps to release that trauma that lives in your bones and in your muscles, your body.

This creative work of grief is one of the major influencing factors with every piece I've created since. I give voice to, or spotlight, some sort of a social injustice, in every piece KPC creates.

REFLECTIONS

Why do you make your art?

Grief not only comes when someone actually passes physically from this earth. It's much more complicated, more intricate than that. I created different pieces that spoke to the trauma that I was trying to work through. It started out as a personal journey for me to try to get out my feelings, feelings I didn't know how to express in any other way, except through movement. And then that movement became a musical; it became a storytelling moment.

How do you make it?

It's different for each piece depending on the topic and how close it is to me. Sometimes a song will keep coming up. I'm much more interested in using movement to elicit emotion or express emotion, as opposed to the thought that I want to move a certain way. Music has to make me feel something. It's important to me that the movement stems from the emotional purpose behind it.

RECOMMENDATIONS

Take a class, whether it's a yoga class, fitness, or dance, or just a stretch or breathing class. People become more mindful when using movement as a pathway to healing. But not always.

You might just need to be physically exhausted to expel the emotions, the tension. Movement can take your mind off the present situation.

Focus on your breath. That's all you need to do—just breathe right now. You don't need to do anything else. You don't need to be always mindful and always aware. Give yourself some great affirmations. Give yourself some space. There's no rule book. There's no prescription for the different forms of grief that each of us experience.

Artist: Brad Wolfe (of Brad Wolfe and the Moon)
Art: Singer, Songwriter
REMEMBERING—BRAD'S GRIEF STORY

Grief has been part of my life since as long as I can remember. My grandparents, on my father's side, were both prisoners in Auschwitz during World War II. I heard stories of their lives from as far back as my memory goes.

My grandfather's job while in Auschwitz for four years was to actually help build the camp itself, as part of what was known as the Sonderkommandos—a group of Jewish prisoners forced to perform a variety of duties tied to the gas chambers and crematoria of the Nazi camp system. They were usually killed after a few months and replaced by new arrivals. One of his specific duties was to carry the bodies to and from the crematorium. So many lives lost. He stayed alive by eating the morsels of food he found in the pockets of those who died. The fact that he survived the entire experience is beyond extraordinary.

My grandmother is actually still alive, age 101. Her dad was killed in the ghetto. Her mom was killed right in front of her at Auschwitz, as a guard hit her over the head with a shovel and dragged her away. Throughout the war, she protected her two younger sisters.

Knowing my grandparents' stories made me question so much about humanity from a very young age. I wondered: why do we treat people the way that we do? And what's the purpose of treating people so horribly when life is short?

My grandmother was interviewed over 20 years ago by Steven Spielberg's organization, the Shoah Foundation, as part of research for *Schindler's List*. In her interview testimony, which I only recently uncovered stashed away in the archives at USC Library, the very last thing she says after three hours of recording is: "We should be tolerant of other religions and other races, because we're only here on this earth for a short while." Coincidentally—or not—that had already become my own life philosophy.

As a young person, I was abnormally afraid of death. I felt alone with all these stories and questions, and I felt removed from what I considered to be the "normal" psychological development of a child. And then, my dear friend Sara, a girl I loved growing up, was diagnosed with a rare form of pediatric cancer when I was in college.

I started taking my guitar to the hospital regularly to play music and sing for her. I already loved music so much. It brought to life my emotions in such a cool way. But now, I was able to see the way that music impacted Sara and her physical symptoms: her pain seemed ameliorated when I played for her.

It was a language through which I could connect to her, and I was so grateful for this connection. The music was the bridge. Sara felt it, too. The music led us to some deep conversations about life and death.

I wrote a song for her called "Sara's Got a Sunbeam," which talks about her dreams in life and the fact that she was a sunbeam in my own life.

She passed away about two years after her diagnosis. Grief provided an opportunity for me to reflect on what mattered most. It gave me permission to follow Sara's inspiration and commit myself not just to music but to what matters most to other people—to pursue one's dreams and to live your life as fully as possible while you're alive. This decision to pursue my art around the power of acknowledging my impermanence changed the whole course of my life.

I started a pediatric cancer foundation in Sara's memory called the Sunbeam Foundation to find cures for rare and underfunded pediatric cancers. I simultaneously launched my first full album and started touring, doing odd jobs on the side to sustain myself.

My music career took off rather quickly. I was headlining some of the biggest venues in San Francisco and playing with artists I had loved growing up. Through the Sunbeam Foundation, I had the opportunity to write some songs for other young people like Sara who were facing mortality through their own cancer diagnoses. I interviewed their friends, family, and teachers. And then I would surprise them with the song at their school as part of an assembly.

In some cases, a child would then pass away. I would be invited to their funeral to reprise the song that I'd written for them. Seeing the outpouring of pain in a community when a child dies, but also seeing the amount of love—and that relationship between love and pain and loss—made me further question why we wait until it's too late to celebrate and honor the people who matter most to us. Why aren't we in that state of connection all the time?

I also realized that the success I was having through my music had less to do with the music itself and more to do with the story behind it. Everything and everyone has a story. A lot of the pain that we inflict on one another is because we don't take the time to understand that we, as humans, all have the same kind of stories. We hide them away and don't take the time to listen and discover what's underneath the surface. Think of how much better life would be if we could ask each other, "Why?" Those stories could help us connect.

As a musician, I didn't know too much about "business," so I went back to business school, received an education in design and strategy, and also studied the science of human emotions. All the while, I kept writing and playing music.

This all led me to where I am today, having created Reimagine, a national nonprofit organization to help people face loss and mortality and channel the hard parts of life into creativity, meaning, and impact. We're finally building a social platform to acknowledge that creativity is a vehicle to transform those difficult parts of life into something that makes life rich, and that by doing so, we can also find healing and flourishing. What I'm working on now, and what is impacting so many thousands and thousands of people, is exactly what my grandma said.

REFLECTIONS

Why do you make your art?

Songs and singing bring so much together: words, melodies, voice, writing, and more. It's a full expression. The act of doing it, of actually performing, is such a mindful activity. It immediately puts me deeply in the present moment. When I sing, I really am doing so much at one time— it's what social psychologists call "flow," where the level of challenge is constantly in equilibrium with the level of skill. I combine all of those things—the words, the melodic elements—and it just feels amazing to have all that flowing through me. There's only one place I can be with it: right here.

How do you make it?

The music comes out in different ways, but I always have music percolating in my brain, 24 hours a day. I honestly sometimes dream a song. I wake up in the middle of the night, get out of bed, and go record the dream melody on my phone. Some of those dreams have ended up on my albums.

Overall, writing music is an alchemizing process. I usually have an instrument, whether it's a guitar or a piano, and I will dabble with something free flowing. I'll just start playing and singing, and, without thinking, something will come out. Whatever emerges spontaneously has an uncanny way of being somehow related to what I'm processing.

As I continue singing melodies and playing chords, it all begins to take shape. As different aspects emerge, it becomes like a great puzzle piece to fit it together. The lyrics are being written out loud, as I'm creating. At some point, when it's getting close enough, I'll finally pull out a pen and a paper, and I'll actually go for it, writing down the words, giving it some structure, and turning it into a fully coherent song. It's a very interesting combination: the music and the words and the way they all start magically interrelating as I get closer and closer to something that feels right.

Sometimes there's a pain that I've experienced, and I want to gain a kind of power over it. I will use music and this process to actively channel that energy into another form. Sitting down with my guitar after something hard and allowing myself space to create, then seeing it all begin to emerge into something new, gives me a sense of empowerment and strength. To see and feel beauty emerge allows me to move forward.

RECOMMENDATIONS

Singing feels good. Period. It doesn't have to be your own original song. Turn on a song that resonates with your emotional experience and sing it with the artist. Sing it out loud. There's something about singing that's so healing, because it's embodied. It's literally in our bodies. Singing the words can also help us process our emotions. The song hits you on a deeper level of relation when you're singing it out loud. It's like a chant or a mantra. It becomes part of you.

It can be a therapeutic exercise to try to write a song. But you don't even need an instrument. You can create a little melody for yourself. Maybe write a few words like a poem and try to sing it out loud in the shower. That's where I do most of my best writing, because it sounds so good in the shower. Yes, shower singing. I recommend that!

There's also just experiencing music by itself. Attend a concert, listen whenever you can. Then try to embody it, maybe by taking a music class or a singing lesson. Sounds can elicit meaning so quickly that even knowing a few chords on a guitar can help bring about some kind of processing or healing. The voice is the first place to start. Because we all have a voice, and you don't need anything else or any new skill to use it.

Even creating a playlist of songs can give you a sense of control and empowerment. Think about the order of the songs. Think about the flow. There's art, power, and healing even in that.

Finally, check out *On Becoming an Artist: Reinventing Yourself through Mindful Creativity* by Ellen J. Langer, Professor of Psychology at Harvard University. Whether you're creating a doodle in your notebook or singing a limerick off key, maybe one you wrote yourself, she helps you see that through the act of creativity, you are channeling energy into that present moment. That's all that really matters—centering on a single moment in time and realizing that with creativity or music flowing through you, you are OK.

I wish to thank the artists who shared their time and stories so that others may see something of their own struggle reflected back. My hope is that the reader begins to trust their immense feelings of grief as part of the process, enabling a desire to channel those feelings into artistic energy.

I believe that art enables people to express their grief while reaching out to others or that art reminds us that we are not alone. Art allows those suffering through loss to show their grief in a way that makes others stop, take notice, and perhaps understand and relate—for who among us has not suffered some form of grief?

As an observer, I do know from the hundreds of conversations I have had with people all around the world since the opening of my first play that when we create art, we remind ourselves of how powerful our mind can be. This powerful feeling may only last for a short while, but if we expand that feeling onto a canvas or in a journal, on a stage or on a scratchpad, it may continue to grow in our heart in a universal way.

References

Centers for Disease Control and Prevention (CDC). (2022). COVID-19 Data from the National Center for Health Statistics. www.cdc.gov/nchs/covid19

Fancourt, Daisy & Finn, Saoirse. (2019). What is the evidence on the role of the arts in improving health and well-being? A scoping review. World Health Organization. Regional Office for Europe. https://apps.who.int/iris/handle/10665/329834

CHAPTER 15

The Flowers of Grief

Topaz Weis

*this hurts
had I known
that loss
would hurt
this much*

*I would have
never loved
opened
my heart,
left
my hometown
taken
that job
that risk
never.*

*I need
an off button
to stop
these feelings
I don't want
to stop
these feelings
because then I
just
feel
numb*

good grief
I hate waking
can't I
just sleep
until I
forget
let go
move on
whatever defines me
no longer
a walking
zombie

please
I can't
forget
don't want
to let go,
to move on

but I do
no I don't
want this
grieving
this ending

there is
no end
to this
dark
tunnel

This poem offers a window into the inner landscape of loss that inspired me to design a workshop which I have named "Good Grief, Exploring the Art of Grieving."

Although grief is a human experience that affects everyone on a daily basis, the dominant Western culture doesn't like to talk much about loss and grief. Unless we are part of a religious community, many of us who live in or have been raised by the dominant culture have no dedicated rituals or practices to help ourselves or community members move through times of loss and grief. There is little to no social holding of the emotional pain brought on by loss, and thus many feel isolated and alone. Grief is stuffed down into the body rather than given free expression, and we are left to carry unacknowledged and unexpressed knots of grief in the cellular memory of our bodies, and especially in our hearts.

Grief has a way of sneaking up on us or landing like an unexpected safe falling from a high window. Whether we saw it coming or not, it can flatten us on the asphalt. Any significant change in our life, even a change for the better, will manifest as a loss. A loss of what was known and contributed to the definition of our identity. Some losses are so small that we can easily overlook them; others stop us in our tracks and leave us permanently altered. If life is a series of changes strung together, then so, too, our lives are defined in part by a chain of losses. The resultant emotional state of living with loss is grief.

When a seemingly insignificant loss unexpectedly results in feelings of deep grief for my clients, friends, and workshop participants, I often hear them make statements such as "I don't understand why this is affecting me so strongly. It's not like we were that close." Or when a change is actually a change for the better, but still the accompanying feeling is one of depression rather than elation, people often try to reason away the validity of their feelings of grief with comments like "I didn't even like that job" or "This has been a great move for me and my family. We wanted to relocate. Why am I feeling so depressed?"

There is a tendency in the dominant culture of the Western world to try to reason away grief. As if there is some rational cure for the sandstorm of irrational feelings that emerge uninvited. When we experience deep sorrow over the death of elderly people, many will say, "He was old and sick. He lived a good, full life. So why does every little thing make me cry these days?" As if having had a good, long life should be solace enough for those who are left behind. As if the impulsive reaching for the phone to share a great story with a loved one who will never again be able to answer the phone is somehow a betrayal of the rational mind who knows this joyful sharing will never happen again.

If grief had a color and we could look with x-ray vision at humanity walking down the street, how much of our body's mass would be colored in grief? How many unacknowledged, unprocessed losses piling up, one on top of the other, might be packed into our joints, our muscles, our organs? How much of the air capacity of our lungs might be taken up with the unresolved grief? How much of the heart's ability to feel joy might be suppressed by the weight of sadness?

As the compounded emotional pain of losses never expressed fills our bodies, how can we experience a full range of emotion or movement? How can we possibly have a clear connection from our hearts to our minds when our neurologic pathways are clogged by grief? If this inquiry catches your curiosity, grab some paper, markers, or colored pencils and take a few minutes to intuitively draw an x-ray self-portrait of your body. Now color in the places you have stored your unresolved grief. Then take a few more moments to witness your self-portrait and journal a bit about what you see and experience in your body when you look at what you have created. You might want to have a box of tissues handy.

Not only do our bodies have a backlog of unresolved grief, but we also have seasons or times of the year which hold supercharged grief anniversaries. These are times when our dormant grief wakes up and tries to get our attention. If we are unaware that a grief anniversary is on the horizon, the universe will sometimes provide experiences of absentminded little or not so little accidents and inconveniences to try to get our attention or give us an opportunity to release some grief. We may be taken unaware by an unexplained wave of emotion. The emotional wave can manifest as feelings of tiredness, or an unprovoked need to cry. We may feel agitated or grumpy, or unexpectedly lash out in anger. Often, we feel exhausted and need to sleep for no real reason or our bodies may be hyper-charged and we can't sleep at all.

The body's awareness of the upcoming anniversary is different for everyone and can change for any one person from year to year. If we are aware that an anniversary is on the horizon, we can make the necessary preparations to be able to attend to our emotions during that time. We can, in effect, schedule downtime into our calendar and create rituals to honor our losses. If we can make time for the luxury of grieving losses that have not been integrated or resolved, we can chip away at the process of releasing the grief that blocks us from being able to have a full experience of joy.

Good Grief offers a space to honor our feelings of loss and grief through engagement in the expressive arts. The workshop meets once a week for a three-hour session over a four-week period. Each week, participants are led through an intermodal process of art making. Intermodal refers to the layering of two or more expressive art modalities. The group doesn't spend a lot of time sharing the storyline details of our losses. We all know our own stories and telling them to ourselves and other people reinforces what we think we know about them. In my experience, talking is not the most effective way to transform how we experience our grief or necessarily the best way to release it. Rather, we engage in embodied experiences of expressing from the inside out. Good Grief incorporates the themes of loss and grief into processes which thread multiple art modalities: visual art, movement, and music together with written and spoken word. Art making helps to bring the grief we hold inside out into the light of day where it can be witnessed from a distance. It offers a language for experiences and feelings that are hard to express in words. When our grief is overwhelming or confusing, the arts are useful tools to give that grief a form and life outside of our bodies. Some of the emerging content may be very familiar and some content can be quite surprising.

There is no requirement to be skilled or experienced in any of the arts modalities. I work with a low skill/high sensitivity model that invites free expression without judgment. Each week offers a different process that culminates in a project that can be taken home. Flowers of Grief are one of the beginning projects.

The Flowers of Grief exercise starts with some relaxing breath work and a guided meditation.

I will offer an abridged version of the meditation here.

Find a comfortable position to sit or lie down. You can close your eyes or just assume a lowered gaze so that you don't get distracted by the visual world. Take a few nice relaxing breaths.

Notice how your body expands with the inhale, and on the exhale, see if you can begin to let go of anything that you may be holding that does not serve you. Breathing in and receiving, breathing out and releasing. Take a few moments to let your body become heavy. When you feel in a calm state of mind, I'd like to invite you to imagine a beautiful space where only helpful influences can enter. This can be a place that you have been to before or somewhere made up from your imagination. Take a moment to open your senses and explore this beautiful space. Once you feel comfortable here, use your imagination to see a path that lies ahead of you. I invite you to journey along that path until you get to a doorway. When you open the door, you will see that you are in a large cave with a long staircase descending deep into the earth. Walk through the doorway and take the stairs down, down, down. At the base of the stairs is a welcoming pool of warm water. There is a magical sensation of peace and total relaxation here. The pool calls to you and you immerse your whole body into the water and begin to float. Know that while you are floating here, all of your needs are being met. When you are hungry, you are fed; when you are tired, you sleep. You have no need for anything here. There are no worries or cares to distract you from the deep peace that surrounds you. There is just the sound of your own beating heart attuned with the heartbeat of the earth. Allow yourself to explore the edges of the pool.

You can dive under the water and, surprise, you can breathe under the water. Such peace and tranquility are yours and it feels as if you could go on forever in this way.

As you breathe in and breathe out, floating in a warm pool deep in the earth, you notice that the pool seems to be getting smaller, or perhaps you are getting bigger. You are now held comfortably but firmly by the walls of the pool in which you float. Where once the water was calm, it is now beginning to shift, and the walls of the pool are vibrating. The walls of the cave itself begin to move closer until your body is so snugly held by the earth that you can no longer move. You are now tightly packed into the space, and the walls are pushing in upon you in rhythmic intervals. You are becoming ever tighter, but just above the crown of your head, you notice there is a small opening. Not much bigger than a keyhole, but seeing as you have nowhere else to go, you begin to reach your head towards that opening in the hope that by pushing out, you will find more space. So you push and reach through the crown of your head until you find yourself in a tunnel. The walls of the tunnel assist you as you reach and push towards the unknown. Push, reach, rest. Push, reach, rest. Then, suddenly, the walls of the tunnel expel you out into light. You feel a waft of air over your face and into your lungs. There is light and sound and smells. The cave and the pool are gone, and you have entered a new world.

Apparently, the pool in the earth is a mother's womb and this meditation is a rebirthing of sorts. Whether we were celebrated upon our arrival into the new world or ignored, birth is, for us all, our first big loss. We are forcibly relocated from a familiar warm, dark, moist world into a cold world of light and air. For some, this transition may be a painful experience. For others, the birth process may feel like a great relief. A participant's experience of the birthing part of the meditation cannot be predicted. It is informed by what a person believes they know or has been told about their own birth story. It can be reflective of a birth story they lived or witnessed, one they know of or perhaps a re-enactment of the birth story stored in their cellular memory. In any case, what came before is forever lost and the baby must adjust to a whole new experience. If the baby is held, fed, and permitted to cry, perhaps some or all of the tension of this primary loss can be released.

The meditation then metaphorically moves through the developmental stages of growing physically, emotionally, intellectually, and socially. Each stage has the repeating idea that once you feel rooted with a solid understanding of your place in the world and your role in it, circumstances change and the pull and push of life propels you onward. As the meditation continues, participants have reported memories of different times of their lives flash into their minds. Some they remember well and some they had completely forgotten about. They see highlights and lowlights. What is important in the moment will find its way to their consciousness. At the end of the meditation, the participants are given paper and pastels to attempt to capture in image form what feels important to remember about the meditation. The group is then divided into dyads or triads to share their reflections of the process and anything else that stands out as important. After this sharing and a short break, I hand each person a Personal Loss Inventory to be filled out.

The Personal Loss Inventory is a worksheet that offers participants a place to record every significant change or loss that has occurred in their life starting with their birth. From the loss of a favorite stuffed animal or having to give up a beloved pacifier to moving households or having a friend move away. I encourage people to write down the deaths of friends, family, and community members, transitions like leaving one level of school to another or moving to a different school building.

Childhood losses like losing a best friend or changes in friend groups are usually prevalent, as are going away to college, job changes, break-ups, leaving your church or religious order for a new path. No loss is too small or insignificant to be chronicled. The ring that your mother gave you that was lost and never found, the broken favorite teacup, and the car accident are all very important to document. The seemingly smaller losses are often quite telling when we look to see in which season the loss took place.

I encourage people to leave space and write in pencil as they are working through their timeline as they inevitably will remember events that preceded the others they have written down. It is amazing what you remember once you start to write down *all* of your life's loss history. Eventually, most people will notice that there is a pattern in the seasons when loss is most prevalent and seasons that appear to be less scathed by loss. This is valuable information that can help with self-care strategies for attending to unresolved grief. When we know the seasons that hold our most significant losses, we can make sure not to overbook ourselves and create more time for reflection and, perhaps, art making.

The Personal Loss Inventory

The Inventory is organized on an Excel spreadsheet with columns for the following:

- Name and brief description of loss.
- Participant age and year when the loss occurred.
- Season when loss occurred (exact date if you can remember).
- There is a column to document what good thing, if any, came out of this experience of loss. It is from our most wounded places that our most profound wisdom is harvested. I believe it is important to find the "silver linings"—the important strengths, skills, and wisdom that emerge from the fertile darkness of the grief lands. An example of a "silver lining" might be when a person's best friend moved away in elementary school, and they became better versed in making new friends and became a good letter writer. Or the break-up of a significant love relationship, which ultimately taught valuable lessons about self-worth and helped identify healthy relationship standards and boundaries.
- The final column documents the "Resolved Grief Rating System." I suggest using a number scale 0–5 to represent how resolved or unresolved the participant feels they are in relation to each loss:
  - 0 = fully grieved, no emotional baggage
  - 5 = never grieved, still very strong emotions when thought about.

  The numbers in between stand for varying levels of loss acknowledgment and grief processing. People can decide what number feels correct for themselves in the moment.

- Multiply the total number of entries in the inventory by 5 to find your Maximum Grief Potential (MGP).
- Add all of the numbers from this column to get the total percentage of unresolved grief carried into the present.
- Subtract the total from the MGP. The remaining number gives a sense of how much grief has been attended to and how much unresolved grief the participant is currently holding.

In and of itself, the Personal Loss Inventory is profound and can be utilized in a variety of ways. For the purposes of this workshop, it sheds light on our seasonal cycles of grief anniversaries and the content that informs the different layers of the Flower of Grief.

How to Make a Flower of Grief

Materials List
- Four pieces of 8" x 8" watercolor paper
- Watercolors with paintbrushes
- Metallic pens, ballpoint pens
- Toothpicks
- Glue (Elmer's is fine).

Instructions
Basic paper rose craft directions for making these flowers can be found all over the internet and on YouTube. Here are the basic instructions with my embellishments.

- Take one square piece of paper and fold it diagonally. Make two more diagonal folds to create a small triangle.
- Open the folds to see each of the four whole pages of paper. Cut along the fold lines and remove one segment from the first piece of paper. Take the second piece of paper; cut and remove two segments from it. Cut three segments out of the third and cut four segments out of the last piece of paper.
- The open edges of each paper will eventually be glued together and will be nested together with the smallest one segment piece being rolled and glued in on itself, resting in the middle of the flower.

- The flower grows by layer with the next layer being made with the section containing two segments, then three segments, and so on until the largest piece of paper creates the outermost layer of petals (see photo below).

I use the creation of the Flower of Grief as a metaphor for the excruciating beauty of the grief we hold in our bodies and experience in our hearts. The flower design uses a process of layering to hold the participant's layered experience of grief. The template is the same for everyone, but people personalize the style by making the shape and color of the petals with their own unique mark. Petals can be smooth and rounded, spiky, feathered, or even frazzled on the edges. I encourage participants not to overthink the shapes or colors they choose but to let themselves be intuitively guided. I encourage them to allow the flower to decide its own shape and colors, and to be open to being surprised at how the flower wants to show up. In the expressive arts field, we believe that once a work of art is created, it is its own entity. It is not a reflection and magnification of the artist's inside self, though it may share some similarities with its creator because she or he is the vehicle through which it has become manifest. Instead, each creation is its own entity with its own voice and story. The final product becomes a walk-in of sorts who has come to have a conversation with the artist and anyone else who wishes to engage with it.

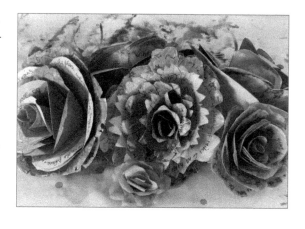

Skilled artists and novices alike will both tend to want to control the outcome of their creations. Having a set idea about what the flower *should* look like in this workshop tends to be a set-up for frustration and disappointment. At best, this process is a collaboration between the artist and the flower, working together to birth and build its form. Some of the raw materials come from the artist's personal experience of grief. But for the actual form and look of the flower, I encourage the participants to use their imaginations to talk with their flowers as they are being made. Ask the flower these questions below and listen deeply to hear the answers. Write the conversation in your journal or just jot down a few key words. For some this is a literal conversation that can be journaled, for others, it is a purely intuitive process.

Questions to Ask the Flower
- What shape are your petals?
- Are you multicolored, two-toned, or monochromatic?
- Which colors belong on which of your layers?
- What colors and words can be seen and which are hidden?

The information on the Personal Loss Inventory is designed to inform what gets written on the petals. I had originally thought that people would choose to write the names and events of their most significant and insignificant losses on the petals. I guided them to check in with themselves about which losses belong hidden on the inside or on the backs of the petals and which could be placed in plain view.

I could not predict what types of losses people would put where. It has been fascinating to witness the choices that have been made around what is seen and shared and what is tucked away or blotted out or written in code. What I learned from my groups that really surprised me was that many people chose to write the contents of the "silver linings" column all over their flowers. For many, these flowers became beautiful touchstones of hope and resilience rather than a container to hold their losses. Many shared with their group that the majority of what they wrote on the petals was the learning they had cultivated from reviewing their loss history and the positive messages that the flower had shared with them in their conversations throughout the process. By the end, everyone has bonded with their flower. A special relationship develops where people feel as if they have made themselves a friend.

The process is not without its frustrations, and everyone feels challenged at some part of this crafting experience. Whether it is in the cutting, the painting, or the gluing, the process of building the flower can take a person to the illusory walls of judgments that they tell themselves. The whole enactment is a metaphor, and I encourage everyone to employ magical thinking and address each obstacle that arises as medicine to help them on their journey. I encourage them to continue to communicate with the flower throughout the process, to listen deeply, with a sense of humor, to what the flower has to say. Some flowers can be persnickety, so a good dose of fake-it-till-you-make-it may be called for. At all times trust the process and know that it is the process not the product that is most important.

Once the paint and glue on the flowers has all been dried and the writing is where it feels it belongs on the petals, there is time to journal reflections about the process and anything of importance that wants to be acknowledged. We then come together and circle up for an honoring ritual. Each participant breathes life into their flower, cupped in their two hands. We introduce our flowers to the group and talk about the poignancy of such beautiful flowers coming out of a lifetime of loss and grief. We share the wisdom that has emerged from the process. Ironically, there is usually a lot of laughter in the sharing. Participants say that the making of the Flower of Grief took a giant weight off their chest. They shared that honoring their losses helps them to feel clearer, lighter, and more aware of things that they need to attend to in order to free up more space in their lives for joy.

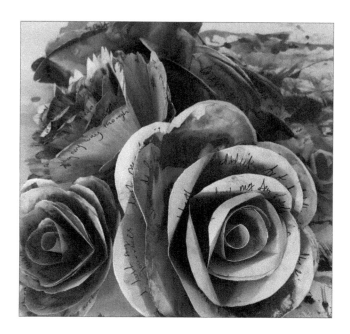

PART FOUR

SUMMER

In Fullness

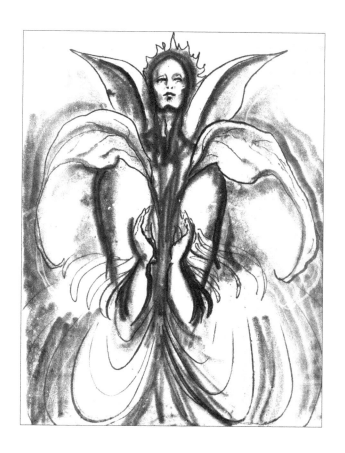

Painter Dad

I feel my father painting the sky,
broad-stroke blues overlapped
by sponging orange flames
setting west.

A man so stoked by image,
his soul reflected in the natural world
melding both together,
signaling remembrance.

An icon of his art,
in my heart, his voice in my ears
sometimes my tears.
I miss him.

Wishing I could continue
to tell him, though I did,
which finally,
must be enough.

~ Deborah Mesibov

Summer Reflection

Claudia Coenen

In summer, everything is in full bloom and energized. The heat of the sun burnishes our skin and we splash in lakes, rivers, pools and oceans, delighting in the feel of the cool water. Sitting by the sea, the waves crashing ashore are like waves of grief, the receding water a reminder that the grief waves pass. The sea swells and crashes again, lapping the shore, erasing any footprints or sandcastles that hug the tide line.

> From time to time, a big wave of sorrow might hit—sometimes out of the blue. It can be disconcerting to feel such intense feelings again. The waves are part of a long-term healing process; they will continue to come and go. Don't talk yourself out of this experience; fully embrace the feelings that surface. (Kennedy, 2014)

In our grief, we are touched on every level of being. Our emotional response is the most obvious, but grief affects our capacity to concentrate, to think clearly, to remember what we are doing. We might have trouble sleeping through the night, or we may find ourselves longing to sleep all day long and during the night too. Our ability and desire to eat, to take care of our bodies, takes a hit as well. This grief is not ours alone, although our life might be the most affected; the death of someone also has an impact on family, friends and the community at large. Death raises philosophical questions that touch upon spirituality and our sense of who we are. When we are able to integrate these five realms of being—the emotional, cognitive, physical, social and spiritual—we bring ourselves into balance as whole humans.

Wholeness seems out of reach in the midst of bereavement but the path towards achieving it is also the path towards living fully again.

Everything that happens to you is flowering you into being.

Reinekke Lengelle (2021)

References

Kennedy, A. (2014). *Honoring Grief: Creating a Space to Let Yourself Heal.* Oakland, CA: New Harbinger Publishers.

Lengelle, R. (2021). *Writing the Self in Bereavement: A Story of Love, Spousal Loss, and Resilience.* New York, NY: Routledge.

CHAPTER 16

Hundreds of Tiny Rocks

Louise Allen

Introduction

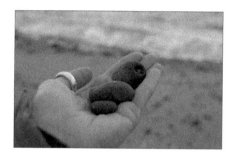

Grasping for a transitional movement-based metaphor to tie together our inner world of grief with the season of summer, I felt a tiny panic rise in me. As I looked to nature for inspiration and a deeper insight into our inner world, my first, fleeting thoughts were "But it's so still. No noticeable change is *happening*. How can I connect this to the loss in grief?" I observed the flowers in bloom and the leaves open and unfurled. I saw an abundance of food sources, of summer fruits and vegetables, long past the losing and decaying and reabsorbing of autumn and winter. Everything is in completion, or fullness. I wondered whether this is what I should or wanted to explore here; the places in grief where there is a sense of completion, of coming to a resting place or acceptance. A sense of ripeness within the grief process.

Of our ecosystem, we do not only have living beings that can embody stillness, but landscapes, weather, the earth, seas and rocks. Stones (beach pebbles) played a formative role in my training as a counsellor several years ago. Our training venue was on the seafront in Lydd, Kent, a few minutes' walk from Dungeness Nature Reserve; a pebble beach surrounding us and the sea ahead. The landscape holding and framing space for a whole palette of skies and seas throughout the two cycles of seasons I was a visitor there. The land seemingly bleak to the unfocused eye and wide-angle lens, flat and bare. Up close, though, many protected species, nesting seabirds, plant life and insects live alongside the shingle. According to the RSPB,[1] it is "the third most biodiverse site in the country for its insects, including a large number of rare bees." The shingle not only provided a habitat for insects and birds, but a habitat for me to reflect and gain a deeper understanding of my own internal biodiversity of thoughts, feelings and experiences. I often walked my feelings over the pebbles while my thoughts whirled in my head. I took in the colours and the shapes, felt the movement under my feet and breathed in the air.

During one training session, our tutor, Nick, invited us onto the beach to choose a stone that represented us. We were to bring it back to the group to share our stone. It was around that time that I excitedly realised that nature could play an integral role in my therapeutic work.

Since then, I have picked up and pocketed countless "treasures" of pebbles that spoke to me. I've rolled hundreds in my hands, scoured the beaches for "the one" that captured what I needed it to. I have pots of stones, little collections with significance and one or two pebbles that I carry with me when I need a touchstone to my heart and soul. These stones are not mine; I borrow from them and take guidance and comfort from them—they're precious to me. Each holds memories, parts of myself or others they represent, and beauty or curiosity. In my therapy room, I always have a bucket of beach stones of different shapes, sizes and colours.

We can explore so much when we work with stones. Our inner experience, the different parts of ourself and our feelings—one part does not negate the other; these different parts coexist just as a round, smooth, brown sandstone pebble does not mean that a whole beach is one round, smooth, brown beach. There are shiny, black and white, chipped flints, too. Dark grey chunks with white quartz lined through, hag stones with holes worn through, broken brick and sea-tumbled glass. Different pebbles may represent different parts of ourself, or the different facets of a pebble may represent the different facets of our grief.

And then there is the opportunity to explore, through stones, how we feel about our place in the world. For example, one pebble may be free to tumble and roll. One pebble may be trapped within a hole in another. There might be one rock lodged under the sand, set apart from the others, with

---

1   Royal Society for the Protection of Birds.

only a small part visible above the surface of the sand. This, too, can open up the space to be curious about how we experience the conditions around us, how we are impacted by others and how we impact the conditions others experience. Pebbles are moved by people's feet, thrown and dislodged by the tide, sometimes picked up and thrown into the sea or used to build walls, pathways, houses and more. Some larger rocks hold others in their dents, worn away by erosion over time.

Working with stones enables us to explore, too, our relatedness to others and how we feel towards the parts of ourselves. We can consider how we feel when we hold, look at or position a stone as we talk about what or who it represents.

If I go back to my initial thought of "everything has already happened," I recognise that this isn't true of nature, of course, just as it isn't true of grief. There isn't a start point and an end point. In nature, the stages of growth are dependent on our species and where we live, the place in the life cycle of each being. In reality, around me in the UK, even in moments of seeming stillness there is a thrum of activity and busy-ness of collecting and making and creating: pollination and photosynthesis, bird song and lawn mowing, chatter and music being played.

Even in the flowering or fruiting, even in the resting or the play, there is an innate continuation towards growth within each being and a transitional interdependence as one opens and gifts, another takes in and the tendency towards something new continues. For example, flowers are opening up to enable pollination, which is necessary to create new seeds and continue the plant's lifecycle. At the same time, the insects pollinating the flowers are taking in food sources to give them the energy to sustain their lives. Other animals may eat the fruits from the plants and so the web of life ripples out. Even with the hard stones on the beach, which seem to be fixed in shape, they will change in place and ever so slowly change in shape and texture in time as they continue to be moved by the tide.

Grief doesn't end with loss, with absence. This is part of grief, but it is not the whole picture. When someone is no longer there, it may feel at times as though this means nothing is there, but actually there is also a space where someone once was. Something new (the space) has been created. We might think of this as winter. And so summer might be considered as the place where something new has grown from and/or into that space. Something that would not have been there in the same way without loss.

A humbling aside was also born from my reflecting—an incidental but valuable flowering in my awareness. I was trying to find the words to convey what I experience as the ease of summer: the comfort of being able to be outdoors without the winter layers for protection and an easiness and opportunity for slowing down, joy and liberation in the warmth of the sun's rays. At the edge of my awareness was an unease in writing this. As I brought my attention to the feeling of unease, I realised that while I was basking and enjoying 20°C (68°F) heat in the UK, several cities in India were experiencing summer temperatures of 42°C (107.5°F), adding layers for shade and skin protection. My unease was a reminder of the importance of being open to understanding the world in which the person we are listening to is living, so we can meet them there in their individual experience with their grief in their present moment. One does not negate the other—my experience of joy and freedom in my summer is just as valid and real as someone's experience of being stifled and threatened by their summer. Likewise, our individual relationship with our own grief can change from one day to another. The life position someone finds themselves in may feel easy and joyful one day and intolerably lonely the next. I understood in this that this truth, this diversity and complexity, is lost when I seek certainty. There is often a tension here that is prevalent in our society—the positioning of our grieving in a hierarchy. The "I shouldn't feel this way when others have it worse" or the "I should be over it by now" or "Shouldn't I be feeling a lot worse than this?"

My observations of nature in summer may also say more of my personal relationship to grief and change, rather than a wider teaching from summer itself. It reminded me of a short blog post I shared on my Instagram account in June 2021:[2]

> After repeatedly ignoring my body's cues calling for some time walking and connecting with the other-than-human world outdoors, I made a choice to prioritise a wander this morning. My head was telling me I shouldn't, there was too much to "do." My body was sluggish and slow and couldn't be bothered, and nowhere was appealing to go to and the weather was grey. And yet I have got to know the fuzziness in my head and body that was also there, a lethargy that feeds itself. And I know that, for me, just taking a step into nature leads to a shift somewhere.

---

2   www.instagram.com/p/CQrTfoHlp4k

I mooched along well-trodden paths and couldn't not notice the beautiful grasses and the fruiting plants in their different stages. I spied hedgerow plants I know to be edible and gathered a few. I slowed to the pace my body had the energy for and noticed a synergy with the physical world around me, the air and the gentle buzzing and the breeze. I discovered a swing in a nook in the trees and let the momentum of my sitting on it do the work. I picked up some litter around the swing, as much as I could carry without a bag to put it in, grateful for the swing and the trees and pleased to be able to reciprocate the care. I collected a few pieces of broken pottery from along the creek, not sure what I'd do with them but feeling the urge to gather nonetheless.

I still felt slow when I got inside, but the fuzziness had lifted and the tension of the "shoulds" had evaporated. Being slow now felt OK and peaceful and valuable.

This post remains one of my most interacted-with posts on my Instagram "grid"; the message resonated with many people and I think this says something of an often-shared experience of thinking, and even feeling, that we *should* be feeling something we are not.

Perhaps we see this in grief, in those moments after a loss, or as we are anticipating a loss, when things do feel OK. Or when things even feel joyful. Or when things are still and we fully feel in the moment with the enormity of whichever feeling arises. Or when years after someone has died, or we have left a relationship or job or home, and we still feel the weight and the sadness of what we no longer have.

Whether we find ourselves assuming how others may experience an aspect of grief or loss, or someone is judging their own experience as "right or wrong," "appropriate or inappropriate," "healthy or unhealthy," I bring it back to Carl Rogers' wisdom—"The curious paradox is that when I accept myself just as I am, I change" (2004). If we can understand the different parts of ourself that are present in that moment, and how they are interacting, and can accept ourselves fully, then we can continue to grow and we psychologically change.

Working with stones as metaphors for these different aspects of our experience helps to deepen our awareness of these parts of ourselves and accept them as they are in the moment. The process reminds me of a blog post I read around the same time as we were invited in our counselling training to choose a stone to represent ourselves:

He talked while I listened and asked a few more questions. When we were done, he told me that some measure of peace had returned. It was a peace that had come from within him, not from anything I'd said. I'd simply helped clear some rubble that blocked his access to his own soul. (Palmer, 2016)

In therapy, we are holding space to get to know those stones that make up the rubble of grief and of life and human experience.

As most people who have embarked on an inner journey of self-discovery and awareness, it is not always easy to be with every part of ourself just as we are. If we take Irvin Yalom's (2011) analogy of "staring at the sun," it can feel too painful, or even be impossible, to directly look at or fully comprehend our own mortality or the mortality of others. Viewing and exploring thoughts, feelings and meaning associated with death through a creative medium can be a way of reducing the glare and perhaps even providing opportunity for greater insight. We can do this by using the liminal space between therapist and client to project onto, or by using metaphor and symbolism through a number of mediums.

When we work outdoors in therapy, we have an abundance of creative prompts in our liminal space. The following technique uses stones, but any natural material can work.

Method

If you are working indoors with stones in the therapy room, establish whether the stones will need to be put back at the end of the session, or if a chosen stone can be taken away if the person wishes.

If working outdoors, establish a shared understanding of whether the person may take a stone from the beach. Although widely done in the UK, the Coast Protection Act (1949) states that in the UK, it is unlawful to take any natural materials like sand and pebbles from the beach, no matter the amount. You can be at fault for taking just one pebble from the beach. This law is in place to protect the natural environment.

Invite the client to consider how they identify in their current moment and to choose a stone that represents them right now.

Invite them to talk about their chosen stone (or other item) and how it represents them.

Then, without interpretation, enquire about the following as seems appropriate:

- How do they feel towards the stone?
- Notice how they hold/move/interact with the stone. Ask if this says something about themselves.
- Is the shape, size, colour, texture significant?
- How was the process of choosing the stone? For example, did they go for it immediately, reject others, were they looking for something in particular... And does this way of choosing how to represent themselves say anything about their inner world?
- What would they like to do with the stone? This question applies both while talking about it and when the session ends.

This can enable the opportunity to connect with their subconscious (through inviting them to consciously choose a stone that represents them) and unconscious (what else is relevant that was not intentional). Some people may not know why they were initially drawn to the stone; some people may consciously have an existing idea of what sort of stone represents them. Either way, the exploration enables a journey and reflection through their conscious and unconscious experience.

As the client projects their inner world onto the stone, they may develop a surprising attachment to the stone. Some people may not want to put the stone down; some may have an urge to throw it into the sea or bury it. Others may discard it easily or not want to look at or hold it too closely. This can often be a rich opportunity for further exploration, so allow plenty of time for this part of the process, inviting the client to consider if and how their relatedness with the stone reflects their relatedness with their experience/identity/part of self/emotion.

This method of exploration can also be used to explore the clients' relationship to the person/thing they are grieving—by choosing a stone (or several) to represent themself, and one to represent the person who has died. Go through the same enquiry as above, and also invite the client to consider:

- Is the proximity of the stones to each other significant?

- Do the similarities/differences in size/colour/shape represent anything?
- Are the different sides/facets of the stones positioned in a way that means something (e.g. a smooth or rough side facing up/down/towards the other, a hole visible or hidden)?

How and When It Can Be Used

In addition to the idea above, this intervention is versatile and can be used briefly as a creative "check in" at the beginning of a session—"choose a stone to represent how you are feeling right now."

It can also be used as a way of capturing the essence of a session or journey—"choose a stone to represent our session today/work together/your journey through grief."

It can be helpful for bringing a new perspective to an experience, or if someone is unsure how they feel or does not know what to say.

References

Palmer, P.J. (2016, April 27). The gift of present, the perils of advice. The On Being Project, April 27. https://onbeing.org/blog/the-gift-of-presence-the-perils-of-advice

Rogers, C. (2004). *On Becoming a Person: A Therapist's View of Psychotherapy*. London: Constable.

Yalom, I.D. (2011). *Staring at the Sun: Being at Peace with Your Own Mortality*. London: Piatkus.

CHAPTER 17

Transformed by Loss

Art Therapy Self-Portraits and the Redefined Self

Sarah Vollmann

Grieving patients in my art therapy practice often instigate the creation of a self-portrait.

Some plan to create an image of self from the outset, while others only recognize themselves in their art pieces after their images are complete. Each portrait is distinct, unfolding with its own form, process, and final product, but the drive to create a self-image seems to be organic and commonly shared in the bereavement treatment process. The self-portraits that have emerged over the years in my office were created with limitless imagination and a range of materials, including collage, paint, clay, drawing supplies, and doll-making materials. For the purpose of this chapter, I am defining self-portraits as representations of self as identified by the artist, to include figurative portraits as well as more abstract and divergent self-representations.

Self-portraiture is utilized to assist and promote treatment in varied clinical disciplines and settings. Many projective drawing tests, such as the house–tree–person or the draw-a-person test, include the depiction of a human figure to assess a patient's self-image and personality, and to elicit unconscious material. Self-portraits can promote self-reflection, introspection, and self-acceptance, and they can allow the artist to become open and receptive to the self (Alter-Muri, 2007). Hanes (2007) believes that clients coping with addiction frequently utilize self-portraits to create a true-to-life representation of the diseased aspects of self, allowing them to face and explore their addictions. Alter-Muri (2007) states that self-portraiture can assist in lessening depression in treatment, as patients can depict and recognize depressed parts of themselves while also realizing that their depression does not constitute their entire identity. Play therapists sometimes encourage children to engage in self-portrait drawings, to foster self-acceptance, self-love, and a sense of empowerment (Cockle, 1994). Several researchers have concluded that a spontaneous frontal self-portrait can often represent a person's need to confront or contend with difficult issues pertaining to their sense of self (Dalley, Rifkind & Terry, 1993; Hammer, 1967; Schaverian, 2013). It is not surprising that bereaved patients might be drawn to the practice of self-portraiture, as it may allow for the exploration and reworking of an altered or shattered sense of self.

When we contend with loss, we often need to examine, reaffirm, or re-define our identities. The death of a loved one is a definitive type of identity loss (Weigert & Hastings, 1977) that can disrupt established life roles, goals, and attachment relationships (Maccallum & Bryant, 2008). Our sense of self is frequently tied into our most important attachments (Bonanno, Papa & O'Neill, 2002) because significant others play an important role in our self-definition (Jakoby, 2015). When a loved one dies, we lose not only that person but also the parts of our identities that are embodied in the identity composed by the relationship to the deceased (Jakoby, 2015; Weigert & Hastings, 1977). Neimeyer (2006) explains that a fundamental process of grieving is to reconstruct meaning, as our sense of self and our sense of the world may be shaken and changed by the death of a loved one. Major losses often disrupt our coherent self-narrative (Neimeyer, Prigerson & Davies, 2002). Neimeyer (2001) elaborates that the grieving process often prompts the shaping of a new life narrative, to integrate the death into our life story and to connect our past and present selves across the biographical rupture caused by loss. The exploration of identity, including the pieces of self altered by loss and the pieces that remain constant, is central in the meaning reconstruction process, and it often includes the reorganization of our identity as a survivor (Gillies & Neimeyer, 2006).

There are countless examples of self-portraiture in art history. Artists have depicted themselves throughout time and across cultures, pointing to an inherent human need to create self-images. One of our earliest existing examples of painting includes a form of self-image. The cave of El Castillo, located in Spain, contains stenciled hands from approximately 39,000 BCE, painted as negative figures in red ochre pigment. Painted handprints have been found in various caves globally as examples of Paleolithic art, including Europe, Patagonia, Borneo, and Timor-Leste. As the artists left their handprints on the cave wall, they marked their presence and left something of themselves to be seen and found. The imprinted hands from so long ago attest to the universal appeal of the creation of an image of self.

As we delve into the rich trove of self-portraits preserved in art history, we can discover numerous artists who created self-portraits in response to grief and loss. German artist Käthe Kollwitz, who lived from 1867 to 1945, explored grief as a central theme in her artwork because of her own extensive history of loss. Her youngest brother died during her childhood. She was devastated to lose her son in World War I, and her grandson in World War II. Davis and Davis (2012) state that the death of Kollwitz's son was the single-most influential event upon her art. They explain that she used art as a vehicle to process her losses, and that grief was the driving force of her work. Kollwitz created more than 100 expressionistic self-portraits over the course of her lifetime as drawings or prints. They are emotionally powerful, honest, and stark renditions of herself, rendered with minimal color, and the brown and gray tones add to their somber quality. Most of her portraits accentuate lines on her face and a grave expression, conveying weariness and sorrow. They aptly explore an identity that was altered by grief, testifying to her anguish and survival.

Frida Kahlo, a Mexican painter who lived from 1907 to 1954, is another artist who created a series of self-portraits. Kahlo experienced significant losses, including death and non-death losses, and explorations of identity, body image, and loss are prevalent in her work. An older brother died before she was born. She contracted polio at the age of six, which caused a permanent limp and bullying from other children. At the age of 18, she was critically injured when a streetcar crashed into the bus that she was riding. She suffered severe injuries, and subsequently endured 32 surgeries, some of which were disastrous. Kahlo lived with chronic pain and physical disabilities for the remainder of her life. She faced additional losses, including an abortion, a miscarriage, and the unfaithfulness of her husband, Diego Rivera. He had several affairs, including one with her sister, causing tremendous heartache for Kahlo and resulting in their divorce. They eventually remarried.

Kahlo's painted self-portraits are often images that depict both her pain and her resilience as a survivor. In "The Broken Column," she depicts herself naked from the waist up, highlighting her wounds. Tears fall from her eyes, and she is painfully held together by nails and straps, while her body is cracked open to reveal her injured spine. The portrait is centered upon her injuries and physical agony, but she stands straight and tall; Watt (2005) reflects that the portrait conveys her double life, depicting both her proud exterior and the pain she holds inside. In another portrait, entitled "The Two Fridas," she paints two versions of herself, shown as two seated figures who hold hands. One wears a white, European-style dress while the other wears a traditional Tehuana dress in an apparent nod to her dual Mexican and German heritage. A vein connects their two hearts, which are visible through their clothing. The Frida in white has a heart that appears to be broken, and she bleeds with a cut vein. Her counterpart in the Tehuana dress has an intact heart and holds an image of Diego Rivera. "The Two Fridas" seems to symbolize her complex and sometimes contradictory experiences of love and loss, of injury, and of perseverance. Lowe (1991) states that Kahlo's self-portraits powerfully integrate her inner self with her public self, to demonstrate that mind–body separation is an irrelevant construct. Watt (2005, p.646) describes Kahlo's self-portraits as "self-affirming," and points out that her paintings often hold dualities, such as the body she had and the body she lost, sadness and joy.

Many grieving patients in my practice have similarly turned to self-portraiture, exploring their self-image as they evolve and grapple with loss. I have used pseudonyms in the following case examples to protect their identities and privacy.

Mia

A young girl, Mia, was referred to me after her infant sibling died. In our third session, she spontaneously began creating an image of her name in bubble letters, and she worked on it for several weeks. While she often moved through art and play with a relatively short attention span, I noticed a shift in her focus with this art piece. She became deeply absorbed, working painstakingly to shape each letter of her name and filling a large page with oversized, slightly crooked bubble letters. After drawing it in pencil, she confidently traced over her work in marker to make the image permanent. She retraced the borders of her letters to make thick, bold lines, and explained that she wanted to make sure that people could easily see and read her name. We reflected together on the importance of being seen, and considered the complexity of getting needed attention when one's parents are upset and grieving.

She decided to decorate the inside of each letter with small drawings.

She filled the first letter with hearts, "because hearts are my favorite," and explained that she was loving. The second letter was adorned with stars of varied sizes. As she drew them, she recollected singing "Twinkle Twinkle Little Star" to her sibling and spoke of her excitement to become a big sister. She added the sun, because "You are my Sunshine" was another favorite song for them. She portrayed her beloved pet fish inside the following letter and created a background to resemble their fish tank. With pride, she described her routine of feeding the fish and cleaning the tank. She also shared memories of holding and wrapping the baby in a blanket, and of being called her "mother's little helper." We reflected on the loss of her cherished caretaking role with the baby and realized that her pet fish seemed to provide a means to maintain a positive identification as a loving caregiver. She added tears falling from the sun and spoke of missing her sibling.

To finish, she drew strong lines emanating from her name, like huge rays of light. Her name seemed to pulsate with power and energy, and slightly resembled the emphasized lettering in a superhero comic book. She expressed pleasure in the final product, and a plan to hang the image in her bedroom. The progression in her art piece, from tentative penciled letters to a bold and colorful final image, pointed to a heightened sense of mastery and control. This image of self demanded to be seen, in a seeming response to the dynamic with her parents who were loving but somewhat unavailable due to their intense mourning. Memories of her sibling and expressions of her grief were embedded into her name, symbolizing her process to incorporate the loss into her life narrative and identity. Her identification as a caregiver, both lost and maintained, was upheld and explored. Thick lines and bright rays of light reinforced her name, and seemed to visually proclaim that she was alive, intact, and unbroken, despite her loss.

Laila

Laila was newly bereaved when I met her. Her spouse, who struggled with addiction, had recently died of an overdose, and she was the one who found him deceased. She was drawn to doll making and had the spontaneous idea to create a "Dammit Doll." She explained that Dammit Dolls are somewhat similar to voodoo dolls, both visually and in practice; they are stuffed, cloth dolls with a designed purpose of being slammed or thrown around as an outlet for stress and aggression. Laila stated that she wanted a Dammit Doll to throw because of her anger, and she enthusiastically gathered materials to begin creating. The rhythmic act of sewing and binding fabric together seemed to be soothing for her.

As we worked together, Laila repeatedly referenced an altered sense of self, saying that she felt like a different person since her husband's death. She had significantly changed her appearance after he died in an expression of her shifted identity, dyeing her hair a different color and intentionally making other changes in her physical presentation. As her doll evolved, she expressed surprise upon realizing that it looked just like her, and that it had unintentionally become an image of self. She concluded that it could not be a Dammit Doll as planned, because she did not want to throw or slam herself around. She instead designed two sides of her doll to illustrate different pieces of her identity and experience. The first side represented her "good days." Superhero emblems, fireflies, flowers, and apples symbolized her identity as a school counselor, actress, and compassionate person, and her sense of self as a strong, empowered superhero. Sugar skulls were added for her growing acceptance of death and loss. She chose to have the doll's feet facing forward on this side as she decided that this part of herself was moving forward. The second side represented her "bad days." Laila adhered more superhero symbols as she discussed her struggle, on bad days, to find her superhero strength. She explained that rage was the primary emotion for this side of the doll, as expressed through images of the Hulk and a fist, and that the doll's feet faced backwards to symbolize her experience of feeling held back by her grief. She placed a sugar skull on both faces of her two-sided doll. Their placement, like masks over her face, seemed to illustrate the looming impact of loss upon her identity, as well as her attempts to accept and integrate the loss into her life story.

Laila decided to create a little Dammit Doll for her self-portrait doll, pointing to the anger that still needed a vessel. Her Dammit Doll was small and unclothed, and she tied string around its wrists and ankles in an apparent expression of entrapment and suffering. The doll seemed to portray an experience of loss, scarring, and survivorship. Dark stitches formed a vertical line across the doll's body, as if it were once torn in two but then mended. One eye was a black button while the other eye seemed to be missing, with only a stitched, red X in its place. A heart adorned the chest. Together, the two dolls looked like mother and child, and the Dammit Doll seemed to illustrate the anger and loss that Laila carried with her.

As we looked at the two dolls together, we reflected upon the Dammit Doll's role of giving form to her anger and of externalizing a bit of her rage. She mused that while her anger was still carried with her, part of it was now expressed and held outside of her body, providing some relief, space, and perspective. In a surprising twist, we noted that the two sides of her self-portrait doll looked remarkably similar. We speculated that the doll expressed the beginnings of an integration of the loss, of "good" and "bad," and of her shifted sense of self. She subsequently added jewels and lotus flowers to represent the body adornments and tattoos that she had gained since her husband's death. She revealed that the lotus flowers represented beauty coming from dark places. With care, she wrapped a string of beaded words around the doll as positive affirmations, including the words "gentle, feel, live, friend, kiss, learn, and laugh." Her words of affirmation, in tandem with the jewels and flowers, seemed to serve as a blessing for the doll, and for herself in her journey forward. To finish, she tied a silver ribbon around the doll's waist to symbolize the silver linings of her experience.

Emily

I began working with Emily, a teenager, a few months after her mother died in a car accident. Emily was initially quiet and withdrawn in our sessions, but she immediately gravitated towards the art supplies, and they seemed to increase her comfort level. I began making art alongside her as I sensed that our non-verbal immersion in the creative process fostered safety and the gentle building of a rapport. She eventually decided to create a memory box for her mother, but she felt unable to work on the box's inside and kept it firmly shut. This seemed to illustrate her need to pace herself, and to protect herself from delving too quickly or deeply into overwhelming feelings. I supported her choices and pace and followed her lead. For many months, she painted the top of her wood box. As it was shallow, she decided that it could be hung and displayed on the wall like a painting, and it became a poignant self-portrait. She worked very slowly and carefully, drawing first in pencil and then painting with tiny brushes. Her careful and almost perfectionistic tendencies pointed to underlying needs for control. We reflected on the lack of control that we have when a loved one dies, and upon the inherently human need to have some semblance of power in our lives. Her slow painting process seemed to provide satisfaction and a sense of control and mastery.

She depicted a nighttime landscape. A ring of mountains surrounded a deep blue lake, which was illuminated by a crescent moon. The nighttime sky was filled with dark clouds. She placed herself in the left corner, with her back to the viewer, as a small seated figure contemplating the waters in front of her. The figure was expressive and mysterious, her face hidden from the viewer. As with the tightly closed box, pieces of Emily's grief and identity were seemingly unready to be starkly revealed and in need of gentleness and protection. In her creative process, Emily was able to control how much was seen and how much was hidden, and to offer her self-portrait the protection of a turned back and dark skies. The figure was markedly alone and small in the open landscape.

Emily spent many sessions fine-tuning her portrait, repeatedly adding depth and color to the water and brushing in tiny highlights of color. She painted the figure last, seemingly hesitant to fill it in with color and to give full and final expression to her self-image. She carefully painted the hair of the small figure to match her own, dressed her in black clothing, and shared that the dark dress was chosen to reflect her state of mourning. She finally declared that her art piece was complete. Like the painted figure, she gazed into her image quietly and with deep contemplation. When asked about her impressions, she reflected upon the painting's portrayal of loneliness and longing, and said that it accurately symbolized her experience. She recognized hope in the portrait as well, explaining that the figure looked out upon beautiful and deep waters, and that there were possibilities ahead, despite her grief. She revealed that her mother was represented in the crescent moon, shining light upon her from afar and encouraging her to move forward.

As we would expect, Laila, Emily, and Mia created self-portraits that were deeply personalized, with dramatically varied art mediums, approaches to treatment and art making, and final products. They each had their own pace, needs, and ways of relating to me as the therapist, and they were able to carve out a process and product that was fitting in their unique grief experiences. The act of creating a self-portrait was transformational for each of them as they explored and reworked identities that were altered by loss. Mia's image of her name paid homage to her sibling with stars and a tearful sun, but also radiated with newly discovered self-confidence and power, and demanded to be seen. Past and present were entwined as her loss, memories, needs, wishes, and accomplishments were held together in a coherent image of self. She emerged as a survivor. Emily's self-portrait, painted on a shut and empty box, aptly expressed the empty space within and her struggle to face her feelings. Her figure of self sat upright, looking sorrowful but undefeated. As the figure's face was turned away from the viewer, she was simultaneously hidden and revealed, mirroring Emily's presentation in sessions with me and demonstrating her underlying needs for protection, pacing, and control. The moonlit landscape symbolized the void of her mother's absence as well as a comforting sense of her presence and their continuing bond. Laila created a doll of self with two sides, as she felt torn between debilitating grief, anger, and her inner strength and resilience. Through her Dammit Doll, she was able to externalize and give shape to her rage without being consumed or defined by it. Her self-portrait explored, contained, and united conflicting pieces of self, promoting integration. A revised life narrative was begun as she embraced post-loss growth and hopes for the future.

Significant loss often prompts a dramatic change in our sense of self and our worldview. Art therapy self-portraiture can assist with meaning reconstruction, allowing us to reimagine our self-image. Self-portraits can hold and give voice to our most painful feelings and experiences while simultaneously recognizing our strengths as survivors. Pre-loss and post-loss identities can be explored, reworked, and joined in one image, promoting integration and continuity in our life stories. As we step into the role of the artist, we reassert agency, owning and reshaping our narrative and sense of self.

References

Alter-Muri, S. (2007). Beyond the face: Art therapy and self-portraiture. *The Arts in Psychotherapy, 34,* 331–339.

Bonanno, G.A., Papa, A. & O'Neill, K. (2002). Loss and human resilience. *Applied & Preventive Psychology, 10,* 193–206. https://doi.org/10.1016/S0962-1849(01)80014-7

Cockle, S. (1994). Healing through art: The self-portrait technique. *International Journal of Play Therapy, 3*(1), 37–55. https://psycnet.apa.org/doi/10.1037/h0089188

Dalley, T., Rifkind, G. & Terry, K. (1993). *Three Voices of Art Therapy: Image, Client, Therapist.* London: Routledge.

Davis, A. & Davis, M.P. (2012). Kaethe Kollwitz's expressions of grief. *Cardiovascular Diagnosis and Therapy, 2*(2), 184–185. https://doi.org/10.3978/j.issn.2223-3652.2012.01.05

Gillies, J. & Neimeyer, R.A. (2006). Loss, grief, and the search for significance: Toward a model of meaning reconstruction in bereavement. *Journal of Constructivist Psychology, 19*(1), 31–65. https://doi.org/10.1080/10720530500311182

Hammer, E. (1967). *The Clinical Application of Projective Drawings.* Springfield, IL: Charles C. Thomas.

Hanes, M.J. (2007). "Face-to face" with addiction: The spontaneous production of self-portraits in art therapy. *Journal of the American Art Therapy Association, 24*(1), 33–36.

Jakoby, N.R. (2015). The self and significant others: Towards a sociology of loss. *Illness, Crisis and Loss*, *23*(2), 129–174. https://doi.org/10.1177/1054137315575843

Lowe, S.M. (1991). *Frida Kahlo*. New York, NY: Universe.

Maccallum, F. & Bryant, R.A. (2008). Self-defining memories in complicated grief. *Behaviour Research and Therapy*, *46*, 1311–1315.

Neimeyer, R.A. (ed.) (2001). *Meaning Reconstruction and the Experience of Loss*. Washington, DC: American Psychological Association.

Neimeyer, R.A. (2006). *Lessons of Loss* (2nd edn). New York, NY: Routledge.

Neimeyer, R.A., Prigerson, H.G. & Davies, B. (2002). Mourning and meaning. *American Behavioral Scientist*, *46*(2), 235–251.

Schaverien, J. (2013). The Scapegoat and the Talisman: Transference in Art Therapy. In T. Dalley, C. Chase, J. Schaverien, F. Weir, D. Halliday, P. Hall & D. Waller (eds) *Images of Art Therapy (Psychology Revivals): New Developments in Theory and Practice*. London: Routledge.

Watt, G. (2005). Frida Kahlo. *The British Journal of General Practice*, *55*(517), 646–647.

Weigert, A.J. & Hastings, R. (1977). Identity loss, family, and social change. *American Journal of Sociology*, *82*(6), 1171–1185.

CHAPTER 18

The Art of Sending Condolence Cards

Topaz Weis

C ondolence correspondences are sometimes written more for the giver than for the receiver. When someone or something goes away forever, everyone connected to them or it will have an experience of loss. Depending on how much of an unprocessed backlog of grief a person is holding, and how closely they were connected to who or what is forever gone, the intensity with which they may write a note of condolence can vary greatly. I like to encourage people to pause and take a moment before mailing a letter or card of sympathy to examine what their true intentions are in what they wrote.

For some, sending sympathy cards is simply a social construct logged under the title "What to do when a friend, family member, or associate experiences a loss." But if the Victorian rules for proper etiquette are not what is motivating you, ask yourself what you hope the card will achieve.

It is important to be clear about your intention and do a bit of your own personal work around the loss before sending your note. Although feeling emotional when you are writing can sometimes help the words to flow and invite the assistance of the Muse to find those perfect phrases, be cautious. Are you writing your note to make yourself feel better or are you writing it to help the recipient feel better? Maybe write a rough draft for yourself first. Use that draft to open the dam on your own river of grief. Give yourself the gift of expressing what you are holding around this loss before you venture to offer sympathy and support to the bereaved. It is all too easy for your own grief to spill onto the page in a manner that can burden the recipient beyond their own experience of loss. Misery only loves company when everyone has the support they need and no one needs to swipe their own grief off the table in service of someone else's. This is especially true when the experience is cloaked in the disguise of offering sympathy.

Also, be authentic and don't worry too much about sounding well versed. Speak from your heart. Most people can easily discern when someone is being sincere, and it is hearing your sincerity that will reach their hearts, no matter how clumsy the presentation.

Some people have a special knack for writing condolence cards and letters. They find a way to express sympathy and give the reader the sense that their experience of loss is recognized. The best condolence cards will leave the reader feeling seen, held, and cared for, as opposed to the worst condolence cards which will simply leave the bereaved reader angry or exasperated. We don't want to leave the recipient with the sense that they need to take care of us, the sender, in any way.

Sending a sympathy letter is different from sending a card. The letter provides a place for honoring more than just the reader's experience. It offers space to focus on honoring who or what was lost. There are often stories and history recalled in the letter. It takes time to write and time to read. A letter is like sitting down to a meal with a grieving friend, whereas the card is more like meeting for tea and cake. The best condolence cards honor the recipient's experience and hopefully leave them with a modicum of hope or some sweetness to savor in the moment and carry into the future.

My Good Grief: Exploring the Art of Grieving workshop culminates in a condolence card project. The process begins with all participants sitting in a circle discussing the worst condolence cards they have ever received.

It is generally agreed upon in this workshop that the cards that venture to tell us how we are feeling, or how we *should* be feeling, are the worst. If you don't really care about the effect your card may have or want to stimulate an anger response in a grieving friend or loved one, try sending one of the Hallmark specials which say things like "Those we loved don't go away, they walk beside us every day" or "Everything happens for a reason." In my experience cards like this tend to just become part of the background noise and numbness experienced by the grief stricken. Above all, never start your correspondence with "I know how you are feeling…"

The truth is, from my body over here, I will never know how you are feeling in your body over there. I can intuit your feelings and maybe come close to an understanding of what you might be experiencing, but in truth I don't know how you feel and to say that I do will only distance me further from the connection that I am hoping to make with you. I can empathize and sympathize. But even if I think I have experienced the same exact thing, it is simply not humanly possible for me to know the depths and nuances of another person's feelings.

Once those of us in the workshop circle have all rolled our eyes, shaken our heads, and had a good gallows-humor laugh about the worst cards, we talk about the best cards we've ever received. We also talk about the types of communication that would have been helpful or at least appreciated at different times with different types of losses. There is no one-size-fits-all when it comes to grief. No two losses are ever the same, and our needs change with each circumstance. It is hard to know what will hit home for any one person, which is why, when creating a condolence correspondence, we must really trust our hearts and be guided by our intuition. It seems odd to write a condolence card to yourself, but if you've never done it, give it a try. I believe you will find, like the participants in my workshops have found, that a lot can be revealed about what your needs are and what kinds of self-care you are requiring by sending yourself a sympathy card.

After our discussion, I lead the group to the materials table and invite them to create the card they would most like to receive in their current situation of loss or from another time of grieving in their lives. I encourage them to allow their needs and feelings to inform their card making.

The Project

You are each invited to create a card which contains words, images, textures, and colors to express what would feel like the perfect message of condolence for yourself. Think about what would be meaningful to you. What would be, or would have been, helpful and healing for you to receive from someone who is sending a message condolence during a specific time of grieving in your life?

Create this card with the knowledge that someone else in the room is going to be taking it home with them when the workshop is over. If your inner critic pops into the room for a visit, thank them for their help but explain that their services will not be needed. I invite you to trust the process wherever it leads you in making this card. If what you make looks like a mess, then make a mess. Grief can certainly be messy, and there is likely someone in here who wouldn't mind being reminded of that. Open yourself to the magic and serendipity that can happen when you allow the creative process to lead the way. I guarantee that the card you make, inspired by what you wish you could receive, will be perfect for someone else in this room. Try not to think too much about the fact that someone else will be receiving this. Allow your heart and the creative process to lead the way. Have fun!

My studio has a virtual mountain of materials. There are bins, boxes, and piles of different papers and yarns, paints, markers, and glitter. Treasure troves of found objects, beads, bells, baubles. Just about everything you could want for creating color and texture, and hot glue guns to effortlessly put them all together.

Giving yourself permission to play is the most important ingredient. I encourage people to allow the materials to choose them. There is a big box of silk flowers and dried flowers. A lot of people like to incorporate flowers into their card designs. Some cards are intended to meet a person in their grief. Other cards attempt to bring laughter and joy. All materials and messages are informed by what the workshop participant would find most helpful and most healing to receive in their own time of grieving. The cards can be meant to be read at face value or as a metaphor. They can go deep into a particular meaning or be kept general and open for interpretation. No rules, no judgments; feel, play, and create is the assignment.

Someone once designed an It's-Time-to-Lighten-Up card drawn on an oversized balloon whose design expanded when inflated by the recipient. Cards have been created with broken pieces of mirror revealing a fractured reflection of the viewer; another had zippers which had hidden messages glued inside. Mostly, though, the cards are simple, made with papers and pens. One card had the message "Rip up this card. It will feel good to destroy something!"

There is a wonderful camaraderie that develops in this workshop, and after three four-hour expressive arts sessions, the group has developed a sweet intimacy. The participants don't often all know each other before the workshop begins, and although we focus primarily on art making, some snippets of people's stories are shared and a blanket of caring shrouds the group by the time this exercise comes around.

As the cards are being made, it is easy for a participant to wonder who will end up with their card and feel a little nervous about it not being artistic enough or being seen as dumb or shallow. All sorts of insecurities can surface. Part of my process in facilitating this is to remind people to send the inner critic out the door whenever they notice that it has come into the room. I keep the energy playful and play music that is calm but uplifting. I check in with each person to see how they are feeling about what they are creating and ask if they have the materials they need or if they need help troubleshooting how to get a desired effect. Most of all, I encourage them to stay focused on creating the card that they would most like to receive and try to not worry about how it will be received by someone else.

When the cards are completed, we clean up the workspace and prepare for the Musical Cards gifting ritual. Each card is sealed in a manila envelope. I shuffle the pile so no one knows which envelope holds whose creation. Next, I tape an envelope to the back of each folding chair.

Playing Musical Cards

Musical Cards is an adaptation of musical chairs, a children's game that begins with one fewer chair than the number of players. Chairs are set up back to back in two rows. The leader controls the music. While the music plays, the players walk around the perimeter of the chairs. When the music stops, everyone must immediately sit in a chair. The person left standing is out. The leader then removes another chair and the game continues until only one person is left. That person is the "winner."

As a child, I was traumatized by playing musical chairs. I wasn't aggressive enough to fight for a chair when the music stopped. I always seemed to get hurt by someone elbowing me out of the way or stepping on my toes so that they could sit in the chair before me. I remember being the odd one out, standing on the periphery of the game feeling sore, both physically and emotionally. To add insult to injury, as people got "out," they had to stand quietly on the sidelines and watch the carnage as the number of chairs dwindled and the line of standing losers slowly grew.

In the Expressive Arts Burlington studio, Musical Cards is played with the envelope-laden chairs placed randomly around the room, and everyone always has a chair to sit on. I turn on great dance music and we dance with abandon. We dance out anything we may be holding that no longer serves us. We dance individually and together as a group, joyfully celebrating in our own individual style of expressing. When the music stops, everyone gets a chair. The next time the music stops, I have moved a random number of chairs to the side of the room where I am standing. These chairs will eventually form a small circle. Once the music stops and a dancer chooses to sit on a chair in the circle, that chair becomes theirs and the taped envelope with the card inside is their prize. The process goes on just long enough for everyone to make the transition out of the focused intensity of the card making. The dancing brings the group together and gives them all a sense of rejuvenation and usually a chance to laugh. When all of the chairs are placed in the small circle and filled with a body, the game is over. No one is "out." Everyone has a prize card nestled in an envelope taped to their chair. Everyone is a winner.

(A note about Musical Cards. My version of this game has morphed over time to its current incarnation. It took some time to figure out how to re-claim the game and figure out how to make it feel equitable. In the earlier incarnations, I made some mistakes and realized that many other people were also traumatized by this game as children. For some, reclaiming the game with different rules has been surprisingly healing.)

I ask the group to decide among themselves who will be the first to open their envelope. When a volunteer steps up, the rest of us give them our full attention. They open their envelope, read the card to themself, read it out loud, and then pass it around for all to see. This can be a tearful process with more than just the receiver feeling the impact of the love and blessings that are contained in each card. One by one, envelopes are opened, cards are read, tears are shed, and gratitude is expressed. Statements like "This card speaks directly to me" or "How is it possible that of all the cards that were made, this is the one that came to me and it is so perfect?" are often spoken. It is a mystery, but everyone gets the card that most directly relates to them. In all of my times offering this workshop, only once did someone receive their own card.

Out of respect for this person's privacy, let's call this participant Mary. Mary is the type of person who likes to connect in a soulful way with other people. She is a deep listener, and people will tell her intimate details of their lives because she is a safe person to speak to. When you are in conversation with her, it is easy to feel that she is very interested in what you have to say and that she cares deeply for you. Mary is a multi-denominational minister whose work at the time of the workshop included running creative arts groups at several nursing homes and elder residences. She helped clients, with whom she had built relationships, to transition between life and death, and she held space for the bereaved family members. Mary spent hours each week holding space for other people's experiences of loss and grief as well as being an integral member of a choir that sang at the bedside of dying hospice patients. Like many people in the helping professions, Mary is capable of being many things to many people, constantly caring for others, needs with calm, clear, compassionate integrity.

During the Good Grief workshop, she had shared that she was also going through some significant changes professionally and personally. It was a time of a lot of questions and not a lot of answers.

During the card-opening ritual, Mary was very excited to see who would receive the card that she had poured so much love into (see above).

The front of the card has three layers of torn, ragged-edged paper glued and sewn into place. There is a ball of yarn with two unraveling strands hanging down over a puddle of silver glitter. The caption reads, "It is OK to Unravel."

When I look at this card, it says to me that I don't have to be perfect with neat, sharp edges. The card speaks of letting my guard down. It says that I don't have to hold it all together and be strong all of the time. It gives me permission to be and feel however I need to be in my grief.

When the card is opened, there are four bracelets which Mary wove for the recipient to wear as grief talismans. The grief talisman is another creative process from the workshop. It is a pin, pendant, or bracelet which you can wear to communicate to the people in your close circle or workplace that you are feeling sad because of your loss but that you are OK. It lets people know that when they see you wearing it, you are experiencing grief and want to be given some space to just feel your feelings. It asks people to please not ask how you are doing, give unsolicited hugs, attempt to distract you, or try to cheer you up. It is a message to well-meaning friends and colleagues that you would like your process to be respected and that you don't need anyone to try to fix it for you.

The inside of Mary's card contains the message "Whatever supports you now, may you feel it and know that I love you."

As each envelope is opened, the group gets a little giddy with excitement. Whose card will be unveiled next? When Mary opened her envelope and pulled out the card, she saw that it was the card she had created. Her initial reaction was one of great disappointment. She expressed that she put so much love into the card and each of the bracelets. She really wanted it to be received by someone else. Her eyes welled up with tears, and although she didn't break down and cry, she looked defeated and maybe even a little angry. The universe didn't choose to gift her card to someone else or give her the gift of someone else's card. Even though the exercise was to design a card informed by what would have been most meaningful to you, she was not happy to be receiving her own card.

The group was a bit destabilized by this turn of events. There was a one-in-twelve chance that someone would get their own card, but no one had anticipated it, not even me. As the facilitator, I was going through the speed-dial mental gymnastics of all 130 ways I could possibly handle the situation. I knew that I needed to trust the process and was wondering what profound thing I was going to say when someone else in the group said to Mary, "Don't you deserve to receive your best loving energy?" Maybe Mary needed to feel worthy of receiving a love as strong as the love she regularly bestowed upon others. She always gave the best of what she had to everyone else. We were gentle with her and encouraged her to receive this great gift from herself. It was a wonderful teaching moment for the group to talk about how easy it can be to care for someone else in their time of need and how difficult it sometimes is to care for ourselves. Although Mary had wanted someone else to wear the bracelets and hear that it is OK to unravel, the card chose to stay and speak with her.

What you've just read above is my memory of what happened. While writing this chapter, I decided to check in with Mary. I wanted to hear in her own words what she remembered about the experience. Remarkably at first, she didn't remember being disappointed about receiving her own card at all. She said:

> I remember that it was so special that I got my own card. I had worked with a lot of nursing homes and a lot of end-of-life care. When I stopped that work, I realized how much grief had loaded up inside of me over the years. Working as a caregiver, seeing so much and having to be the support for others took a toll on me. I knew that I still had loads of grief inside.
>
> I think as a culture, so many people talk about being supported by grace. We try to hold it together and don't allow ourselves to unravel or to grieve fully.
>
> As I sat down to create my card, I remember thinking how many different circumstances in the world and my life hold a similar thread of grief or pain. The card I made had a perfectly spun ball of yarn. As soon as I let a couple of threads down, there was a sort of unraveling. And then the unraveling was just a mess. I was trying to un-spin this tight wad of so many layers of yarn. I remember thinking, "Wow, there are so many unprocessed layers of

grief that I am holding. What a mess." The message I put on the card was that "It's OK to unravel."

I thought it was super interesting that I made the card for someone else, but it was actually the message I needed to hear myself. I don't remember being angry or upset that I got my own card, but it makes total sense. I know myself as someone who loves to give to others. I can imagine that I would have felt angry that I put all this effort into the card for it to only come back to me. Right...why?

I don't remember it, but I'm sure I was disappointed because I have a hard time accepting my own wisdom and supporting myself. I think that is something I continually struggle with. It's a practice learning to support myself. I do remember processing the experience myself in a good way. I had that feeling like, WOW. I remember looking at the card too and acknowledging that I really needed to hear my own message.

Mary still has her card. She has a card box that she often looks through whenever she wants to write a card to someone, which is pretty often. She told me:

The interesting part is, I've come really close to giving the card away. I go through the box a lot and I see it. There have been times when different people have had these really deep things happen. I've pulled it out of the box and been ready to write on it, but I can't give it away yet. There's a part of me that just won't let it go. I've actually been saving it. I still need it for myself.

Time and again as the envelopes are opened, the cards informed by the needs and desires of one participant speak with truth and clarity to the person who receives them. There are universal threads that connect us in our grief. We cannot know another person's experience, but if we speak and create from our hearts, our offerings of sympathy will, at the very least, gently touch the heart of the bereaved recipient of our condolences, if not provide a safe haven where they can feel seen and cared for.

CHAPTER 19

Opening into Grief

The Body as Portal to Self-Love and Connection
Becky Sternal

...the heart breaks and breaks
and lives by breaking.

~ Stanley Kunitz (1971)

With every change, we experience loss, though we do not necessarily experience the feeling of embodied grief. For many of us, the day comes when we suffer a loss so tremendous that we are brought to our knees and do not know how to go on. In our western culture, which prizes high functioning and performance, we are often discouraged from collapsing further, falling apart, and from receiving the co-regulating comfort of touch and support. Rather, we feel pressured at times—masquerading as strength and stoicism—to stand up too soon, far sooner than we are ready. And this can affect not only those of us who are suffering but also our ability to support those in need. Because we have not experienced the cradle of support while grieving, we do not always know how to hold one another in our grief. Our reaction to loss can ignite old places of terror and shame, and our disorientating reaction can touch a fear of judgment in ourselves or others. Through this gauntlet of sadness, pain, and suffering, our loyalty to others, to our original bonding, and to society's seeming commitment to dissociation from pain can disconnect us from our true selves and our real human needs in our greatest time of pain.

Our culture often dishonors grief rather than honors it. We can feel lost and confused, unwell, paralyzed, and stuck, when, in fact, it is our society that is unwell and out of touch with the natural rhythms of living and dying. We do not have the mourning rituals in place to hold one another the way we need to so that we can feel met and be held in our grief. We tend to use grief and loss interchangeably, and they are fundamentally different. Experience has shown me that we need tremendous support to move *toward* and open *to* our grief. While it sounds counterintuitive, we need to welcome grief. Opening to it takes courage and self-compassion and support from others. However, our personal histories of unhealed wounds or trauma are obstacles to reaching our own broken heart and meeting it with self-compassion and love. Fresh loss can trigger all that is unfinished inside of us like a landslide. Getting to our grief, which is pure and profoundly human, is the invitation we all must accept if we wish to recover our lives and our aliveness. It is here that we find a way to move forward. Grief gives value to our lives and shines a light on what truly matters—love. To me, all of psychotherapy or any self-work is grief work—longing to recover something we have lost or never had—and healing our wounds around love.

Giving up Pressure

At the very moment we lose someone deeply precious to us, there can be concurrent energies inside or outside of us that give us a "push" to "do" or "start healing." We bring the assault of "more" into an increasingly toxic environment that stunts recovery rather than cultivates it. Even in loss, the relentless energy of pressure can overtake us: "You aren't doing this right." It is the internal feedback we imagine and project. We are confused by our need for space and privacy as much as our hunger for support and connection. When we lose someone we love, there is no longer anything to do, because there is nothing we can do. Grieving comes in waves and takes as long as it needs to take. Those waves surprise us; they can be unexpected, inexplicable, and sudden. Over time, we learn to meet those waves. At first, they might submerge us but eventually we learn to surf along with them. It is not that it is ever enjoyable, but we can practice a deep connection to these powerful forces of nature. We can recognize that we are on our own unique timetable and in our own new universe. We don't exactly know where they are, and when they'll come, but over time they become our own intuitive calendar and map of the heavens. Sometimes our grieving might take a short time—or a lifetime—to integrate our losses into the fabric of our lives. There is no predictable or acceptable pace. We cannot rush our healing, but society tries to convince us that we can.

It is OK to succumb to the forces of grief. We do not need to prove, man-age, or transform our pain. There is nothing to be solved, only a process to be lived and experienced. We should not feel pressured to set up a foundation, write a book, or settle anything. We can if we want to, and we can have a "no"—these are expressions of our own divine freedom. If we create the space inside of our body, and tend to our feelings and our pain, our pain can be transformed, and our grief can transform us. We will know by our tears that we are opening our hearts, for our tears are the sacred expression of the comingling of pure love and pure grief.

We doubt our body's ability to contain this much pain. Our body can feel like a dangerously unpredictable minefield that we cannot yet trust. Unwit-tingly, in this way we add detrimental insult to injury as we *hold against* the grief in our body, creating tension and constriction (i.e. headaches, digestive issues, back pain). Often we collude with societal pressure to "not feel" be-cause we think it will protect our hearts and numb ourselves against further injury and pain. We think perhaps that it will give us a sense of connection and belonging to the remaining people around us and a sense of control in a powerless world. On the contrary, the pressure that meets our pain is the "second arrow." It can further exile us from our body and keep us out of the flow of life—isolated, confused, and unwell.

Moving out of Dissociation and Blame

When we are broken open by great loss, we are forced out of our dissociation. Our egoic structures are ruptured, as well as the false sense that we are in control. We simply cannot process grief from our heads and thoughts, by approaching our grief as a problem to be solved. Rather, it is a journey that connects our heart and the very core of our body. It has been said that the longest journey we will make in our lives is from our head to our heart. Loss is a catalyst for this journey, and we must trust the wisdom of our bodies to show us the way. We must unleash our five senses, to experience the raw power of nature, and to connect inward in order to connect outward.

To meet our suffering, we also must learn to *expand* into it, rather than contract or move away from it. We may want to blame and shame ourselves and others for losses that could not possibly be all our fault. We do this to avoid dropping into the deep and profound powerlessness that we all live with, and so naturally want to avoid. Feeling our powerlessness can feel messy and frightening at first. We fear that we will never feel powerful again, and that succumbing will become a permanent weakness. With practice and connection, however, we can acknowledge the truth of our powerlessness, which, paradoxically, can help us to feel more grounded and potent. There is a great potency to our grief that comes when we learn to fully recognize and support it.

Grief is a process of sitting inside the wheel of life and being still, in the center of it all, and feeling the earth below and the sky above, and life in us and around us. Contained within this wheel of life are our mind, body, psyche, soul, and spirit. Meeting and supporting our grief initiates us into a deeper journey inward, outward, downward, and upward. This is life in its full dimension. Of course, most of us never wanted this initiation. We never asked to move beyond where we were before and confront unimaginable sadness. Death and loss are life's initiations into a new life, a life we did not ask for, and one in which we must find a way to exist. We can learn to surrender to what exists now, and we can walk a spiritual spiral path to find the grace that lives under the complexity and the sorrow. Tragedy and sorrow are at the essence of any spiritual path and interweave of all of life's energies, painful and beautiful.

Understanding and Knowing Ourselves

In a world where we can make ourselves wrong and live as broken beings, especially after great loss, we must somehow find a way to feel our rightness and wholeness. For many of us before tremendous loss, we may never have felt—knowingly or unknowingly—whole, making the grieving process even more disorienting, confusing, and terrifying. As a somatic psychotherapist, my heart and presence hold the container with my clients as they enter their body and find their own answers. It is an experiential modality that includes my client's lived experience and befriends their body, psyche, soul, and spirit. All my work involves supporting clients to "tend and befriend" their feelings and attune to the "felt sense" (Taylor, 2012) in their bodies at their own pace. The philosopher and psychologist Eugene Gendlin (2007) coined this term *felt sense*, and describes it as a physical experience that combines emotion, awareness, intuition, and embodiment. People experiencing a felt sense feel more in tune with their body and bodily processes, even their own organs and parts. My sense of felt sense is when you can close your eyes, feel the unseen in your body, trust any message you hear, and know.

Fritz and Laura Perls, co-founders of Gestalt Therapy, created a roadmap of human personality and consciousness known as the five layers of neurosis: cliché/phony/game-playing layer, role/phobic layer, impasse layer, implosive layer, and explosive/alive layer (Perls, 1970). These are unsurprisingly nonlinear, and are a series of concentric circles, which represent energetic states of being or experiences. The theory is that we move through these layers all the time, and it is our awareness of where we are in the layers that brings consciousness to our lives and helps us to live in the present moment.

My mentors integrated and broadened the original theory and concepts into their own body of work. Their layers have slightly different names: role layer, impasse layer, death layer, life layer, open-heartedness, and oneness with the universe: touching the divine (Alpert, 2021, pp.130–139). They also included Reichian character structure and Lowenian bioenergetics to bring further embodiment within each of the layers. It is a modality of caring, maturing, and taking responsibility.

In both models, life layer is at the center. Life layer is our life force and our core experience of aliveness. Interestingly, life layer *includes* grief. Initially I was surprised to learn this as it seemed counterintuitive. I had assumed grief would be in death layer, but that was before I really understood grief. To reach grief that lives in life layer, however, we do have to go through death layer. In my practice, I help my clients fully embody their death layer feelings with enough support so they can move into life layer where joy, orgasm, need, rage, and grief live fully inside of our emotional body. When we touch our life layer, we live from our sensuality (embodied heart and grounded power) with a connection to spirit/source/unconditional love energy (or wherever we place our faith).

Role Layer

Role layer is the outermost of the concentric circles. It is the layer where we act in ways we learned to perform to get enough—or divert—attention to survive. This is where we developed the ability to fit into our families—the "good child," the "funny one," the "rebellious one," the "smart one," the "responsible one," the "outcast," the "caring one," or the "one with no needs" (Alpert, 2021). Without consciousness, we contorted ourselves in order to survive. Most of us carry our role layers into adulthood as defaults. We can live our whole lives with these masks on, afraid to be who we really are for fear there will not be acceptance or love for us. Role layer is also the place where we feel righteous and live in the binary of black-and-white thinking in order to avoid judgment or criticism. Our roles are problematic since while once they were adaptive to get bonding, they are now maladaptive and prevent us from being who we really are in the fullness of our humanness.

Impasse Layer

Impasse is the next layer inside, and it is where we can avoid feeling or re-experiencing deeper and authentic experiences of aliveness. Because we are committed to not feeling what lies between us and life layer (namely, death layer), we make ourselves comfortable in impasse. Impasse is the layer of emptiness, nothingness, escapism, idleness, stuckness, and disappearing. Here many of us attempt to maintain our dignity (after abuse), though real dignity lies in recognizing how deeply we matter. Impasse is the layer where our energy stops, and we hide in an attempt to avoid feeling our loss and pain. It is the layer of all addictions, compulsions, tension patterns, negativity, fighting, defeating, self-harm, spacing out, falling asleep/not falling asleep, deflecting, forgetting, joking around, gossiping, or busyness (Alpert, 2021).

All impasse behaviors are an attempt on our part to get to life layer without going through death layer, albeit unsuccessfully. This layer holds our family's strongly held beliefs—"If I cry, I am weak"; "If I have a need, I am needy"; "If I have a no, I am cruel and selfish"; "If I am angry, I will be cruel and violent, or someone will be hurt." Beliefs like these left unchallenged keep us in impasse. This layer occurs when we cannot produce our own support and where outside support is not forthcoming (or it is and we cannot take it in so we have a defeating: "yes, but"). The way out of this layer toward death layer is in coming into the present moment, becoming curious about our deeper emotions and taking responsibility—*response-ability*—for our feelings rather than trying to manipulate people and the environment around us (Perls, 1970).

Death Layer

Death layer comes next and is the trauma layer, the layer of unhealed wounds, the layer of shame, and the feeling of near death. Perls called this layer the implosion layer where energies that are needed for living are frozen (Perls, 1970, p.24). Naturally, we do not want to go there or re-experience the pain. These experiences already happened; our body remembers, and we have an intuitive avoidance to the reoccurrence of pain. Some examples of death layer feelings are unsupported grief, annihilation and fragmentation, abandonment, humiliation, rejection, suffering, craziness, feeling criticized, crushed, sub-missive, manipulated, or used (Alpert, 2021, p.121). The less support we have to live these feelings as experiences (and the support they deserve through love, acceptance, and understanding), the more we organize ourselves away from our aliveness in order to avoid these feelings. In effect, the more we won't feel them, the less we can heal them. To re-experience, ground, and release the death layer feelings from our body is to be able to enter the life layer. It is a place where people will consider taking their lives because they think the pain is too much to bear. This is the hardest and most frightening place to work as a psychotherapist, and yet it is essential. We can work with suicidal energy in the polarity of it, homicidal energy. We can support the feeling, never the action. By doing Perls' chair work, as described later in this chapter, we can break the fusion between the two energies that keeps us stuck in our unresolved grief, despair, and hopelessness.

Life Layer

Life layer is at the very center of the concentric circles. It is the part of the personality in which we experience joy, orgasm, rage, grief, and need. In order to truly inhabit life layer, Perls believes that we have to have all five abilities available—joy, orgasm/ecstasy, rage, sadness/grief, and need; oth-erwise, we are incomplete (Perls, 1970, p.23). "Implosion becomes explosion, compression becomes expression" (Perls, 1970, p.22). That is the journey from death layer to life layer. Imploding in to exploding out. Explosion is not performative but rather a freeing up of energy in the body out of for-merly held constriction. "We cannot have sex without sexual rhythm and movement; we can't grieve without our diaphragm shaking and tears being produced; we can't be joyous without dancing" (Perls, 1970, p.31). This life layer is where we claim our dignity, our potency, our right to be loved, to belong, to be free to fully be ourselves. We have a right to have and embody these pure life emotions and their varied intensities: joy to ecstasy, sadness to deep grief, and anger to rage. The more we can embody these emotions, the more we live in an embodied and alive state. We feel aligned, unencumbered, actualized, and in the flow.

Open-heartedness and Oneness with the Universe—Touching the Divine

My mentors added two more layers, open-heartedness, and oneness with the universe—touching the divine. They describe open-heartedness as a "deeper and purer place of aliveness that comes from an abiding sense of support, appreciation, compassion and love for all of who we are" (Alpert, 2021, p.121). Everything is worthy and acceptable of love here: each moment, each breath, each feeling. We love ourselves fully and appreciate others more fully.

As we support ourselves in this place of open-heartedness, we enter a place of transcendence and oneness with all beings and energies in the universe. This is the place of deepest wisdom and connection to spirit and all of creation beyond space and time. Spirit/source/unconditional love energy is what moves us through the layers.

Healing Loss, Moving Through Impasse and Death Layers Toward Life Layer

As we bring understanding and acceptance for each of our layers, and how we move through them, we come into integration and wholeness. We understand how we lived our childhoods often in the way that we organized ourselves *away* from our center of aliveness for survival, just as our parents did, and their parents, and as far back as our lineage goes. "By continually focusing on how ultimate responsibility for living in our own center is within ourselves, we come to the deepest place of clarity, personal power and ground from which to share with one another" (Alpert, 2021, p.139).

This healing work helps us to know and accept ourselves and helps us to contain our own darkness which we meet in death layer. We learn to fully form ourselves, to recognize our very existence, and speak from our center without blaming others. As we evolve in the acceptance of our own darkness, we can open to an experience of oneness with humanity and all living things. This, in turn, allows us to bring appreciation to all we are, and who others are. We no longer have to split off parts of ourselves to survive, which allows us to confront the darkness that lives in ourselves and others (Alpert, 2021, p.129). We become able to have deeper experiences that bring more satisfaction, contentedness, pleasure, and peace.

After loss, we are shattered, and our fear moves us *away* from our center or life layer. It is through a courageous commitment to ourselves to feel and to take full responsibility for these feelings that moves us back toward our center. There we can find surprising energetic rewards of aliveness we may previously have never known possible! Role and impasse layers are defensive layers. We must honor that the underlying intent of all defenses is self-protection. When we are defensive, however, our energy has risen to our heads, and we are no longer connected to our hearts. We can appear detached or hard and rigid.

Traumatic loss forces us to give up our role layer. We no longer have the energy to pretend that we are OK when we are not OK. We never actually give up our role layer entirely as it is there in the quick exchange of pleasantries with neighbors. Our work, however, is to simply become aware when we are in role layer and to notice what happens to our energy. Typically, role layer is exhausting, and many of us do not even feel how exhausted we are until we are brought to our knees by loss and out of our roles. These traumatic events can actually allow us to reform in vital, life-affirming ways. We can emerge stronger and healthier than ever before.

Loss plunges us into death layer—the layer where our unhealed wounds exist. All that has not yet been processed awaits us in what can feel overwhelming and terrifying. The good news, however, is that we have impasse layer—the layer where we get a break from feeling. We gather resources here too before we can plunge back into death layer. Only, without support, remaining in impasse layer is a place where we feel stuck. We do not get stuck in our grief, rather in the stand-off with grief. We are not yet willing or able to form whatever death layer feeling lies waiting for us underneath impasse. What would we have to feel if we didn't drink the drink or binge-watch the show? What would open up inside of us? Whatever that feeling is, it is the scary maze of feelings that shape death layer. With enough internalized support, we can move out of impasse, through death layer and into life layer.

Awareness of Our Layers

Our awareness of where we are in the layers is where our journey to health and wellness begins. When we can know and name where we are, and we can ground ourselves, even in role layer. In this way, we meet ourselves in our humanity and how acceptable we are. None of us is enlightened and able to constantly live in life layer. Our commitment to our own healing and our awareness is self-care and self-loving. Our awareness allows us to keep returning to our own experience, knowing our parts, and trusting our own perception and truth. Each journey through death layer is its own "dark night of the soul" where our perceived darkness has the potential to be transformed in a sort of transfiguration. We have the possibility of becoming beautiful and beloved to ourselves.

In this work, we have the possibility of healing all the unhealed wounds of our parents and ancestors that we inherited. There are unfinished places in all of us, and the grieving process is a great illuminator of these places. What we do not consciously transform, we unconsciously transmit energetically to our children, just as these unfinished places in our parents were unconsciously transmitted to us. Raising consciousness is the work of grounding our own energies and taking responsibility for the ways we know how to harm ourselves and others. This is the path of non-violence and the path of love. Taking responsibility for our despair, denial, anger, hopelessness, sadness, and depression clears the path for the pure experience of grief and love, and the profundity of the human experience.

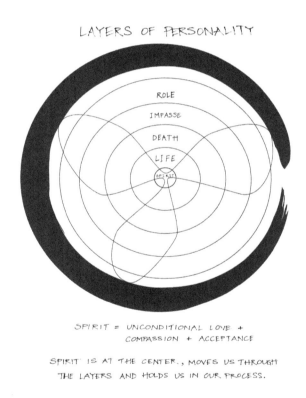

LAYERS OF PERSONALITY

ROLE

IMPASSE

DEATH

LIFE

SPIRIT

SPIRIT = UNCONDITIONAL LOVE + COMPASSION + ACCEPTANCE

SPIRIT IS AT THE CENTER., MOVES US THROUGH THE LAYERS AND HOLDS US IN OUR PROCESS.

Forming the Gestalt Through Our Parts

In sessions, often I will place a pillow in an empty chair directly across from my client. I will ask the client to imagine that the pillow is their heart or broken or grieving heart. I will then ask them to be the energy that comes at their heart that does not let them grieve, or some version of this. Typically, the energy they step into is an energy of judgment, shame, or pressure—or one that tells them what to do, rather than one that could just be with them with compassion. I will then ask the client to embody that energy that does not let them grieve and ask them to feel into their body what it feels like to be this energy. Typically, it is an ungrounded energy that may be afraid for them and trying to protect them, or perhaps it has an "I don't care" in it, or is too dissociated to connect. It is typically also an energy that is disconnected from their heart.

I then will ask the client to switch places and now occupy the previously empty chair where their heart was. I invite them to feel the impact of the energy now across from them. Typically, they will feel emotional, their posture might change, and they can recognize the energy across from them as someone from earlier in their lives. This is where we feel our fear—and our younger selves. I then invite the client to imagine bringing in support and protection. We work in the here and now, as well as there and then; both are fine. For support, some clients bring in their lost loved one, another person—real or imagined, an animal (their dog, a lion or a bear, or an image from nature). For protection, perhaps a client will imagine a wall, a moat, a forcefield, or a bubble around them.

We continue over time to work both sides of the polarity and to bring support in different ways to break any unconscious fusion so they can live these energies more consciously. Describing trauma as being about *frozen* movement, and emotions as being about *fluid* movement, helps clients begin to feel the difference in each chair and on each side of the energy. They can come to recognize that the energies that came at them are now inside of them, preventing them from meeting their own hearts. Owning and taking responsibility for these energies now is an important awareness and powerful part of the work towards healing and integration.

Gentle Initiation Back to the Body

Often my therapeutic process involves a client's gentle reintroduction to their breath and body:

Breath connects you to all of life. Through your breath, you can become aware that you are connected to all that animates our universe. Place your hand on your heart, if you want to, close your eyes, and breathe. Just notice it there with you. Whatever feelings are present, let them be there. Notice that even when you are not conscious of your breath, your body is breathing you. It contracts and expands, like waves gently flowing or crashing, curling forward and receding. Your breath is both constant companion and healer.

When you meet your breath and send your breath to the pain and tension in your body with love, not pressure, you begin to heal yourself. Where your attention goes, your energy flows. Where you place your love, you place your life. Allow your breath to be the unconditional love that meets your brokenheartedness. Become the breath and wave, rising and falling. Like the ensō, feel how your mind is free to let the body create its own circular form moment to moment.

Now, if you can and want to, place your fingers of one hand onto your opposite wrist. Feel your pulse at your wrist. Your pulse is presence. Its rhythm is the drumbeat that connects you to all of your ancestors, and to all of life. If it feels supportive, feel their presence with you now. If that does not feel supportive, perhaps you can feel how your veins are rivers of life flowing into the great river of consciousness to which you are connected— connection going back to the beginning of time. For many of us after great loss, we go into shock and numbness, and our dissociation and disembodiment are protections. Bring appreciation to them. With time, as long as we need, our painful loss can move out of those energetic states and settle into our hearts as pure grief.

Now bring your attention to your broken heart if you want to. With a simple in-breath, gently bring attention to your heart. Feel into your lungs as they fill, and in doing so, feel how they hug your heart with each in-breath. Feel how your diaphragm expands your ribs front to back and side to side. Notice the gentle release of your out-breath. Soft inhale. Soft exhale. In. Out. Notice even the space between the breaths. This moment, this spaciousness, this breath. This simple awareness can be your own renewal. Your own energetic and spiritual cleansing and moving meditation. Do not underestimate the power of your breath. Feel the ever-present symphony that lives in your body.

We heal our heart by being with it. Some Buddhist traditions have a saying that pain is inevitable, but suffering is not. Zen Buddhist Master Thích Nhất

Hành teaches, "If we know how to suffer well, we suffer less" (Hanh, 2013). Being with our suffering, our broken heart, is often easier said than done. For many of us, our learning has not included what it means to be with our hearts and meet all of our feelings with loving kindness, even those that feel intolerable.

Hành believes we have "no birth, and no death, only transformation" (Hanh, 2018). He teaches that the energy of our loved ones takes different forms. We all know life does go on, and it will go on without us one day. Yet, in the moment of traumatic loss, some cannot find any relief in connecting to the greater web of life that holds us all, that connects us beyond the physical realm, while others find great hope and comfort in their faith in an afterlife. Many of us yearn for the physical, naturally, as we should. We are human. That is what we do. We must accept our longing just as we must accept our loss. We cannot have one without the other. Longing and loss. For many that longing directs us to a connection larger than ourselves toward oneness and the divine.

Notice any tension in your body and see if you can move toward it with curiosity. Unsupported grief lives in the body as despair and hopelessness. Unprocessed anger, depression, confusion, shock...all emotions held in the body. These spill over into all our relationships. Chinese medicine believes grief is stored in the lungs and the large intestine. My sense is that it can be stored just about anywhere in the body as tension and chronic pain: as frozen shoulder, back pain, hip pain, knee aches, and overall numbness and tension.

Safety in Connection

Further practices of awareness are mindfulness, or the awareness of "something," and meditation, the awareness of "no-thing." Both practices plant us like gestating seeds in the truth of life. Both help us to hold the polarities and dualities of life that coexist always within us, with awareness as the ultimate container. Evolution and extinction, birth and death, loss and renewal are only few of the infinite polarities we contain. Mindfulness and meditation are important practices for experiencing the fullness of ourselves beyond the binary of right and wrong, and the duality of self and other. We can hold it all. While the practices are deeply supportive and can deepen our connection to ourselves and all living things, they can feel not enough at times.

We also need human connection. We are neurologically wired for empathy and connection on a cellular level. Our emotions and vulnerability allow for this interrelatedness and interdependence. We need to be held energetically—our physical and emotional bodies. We need touch, presence, and caring, and yet, for many of us, we feel alone and unable to trust that there could be safe and supportive connection. We doubt we can have what we need, and that what we need actually exists. Our distrust of others really understanding where we are, and being with us in our pain, often begins in childhood. For many of us, authentic heart connection, or intimacy, was not safe, and we learned to hold against it. Realness and intimacy may not be easy, and perhaps it is our life's work to have enough support inside of ourselves to feel intimate with another human being and meet each other in our grief.

Most of us try to grieve alone, and yet, from a childhood trauma perspective, we were wounded in connection, and we heal in connection. We want the person we love to return so we can feel whole again. Often we do not want to reach out for help, from behind the wall of our pain and sorrow. We just want our loved one to come back. Of course, we would want that. This is so natural. We must, in due time, find a way to reach, and this takes faith and courage. Our grief requires connection to feel supported. "The way out is in," in the words of Thích Nhất Hánh (Hanh, 2015).

Becoming aware of ourselves and our bodies helps pave the pathway toward an ever-present and ever-deepening connection and intimacy with ourselves and others. This is the nature of true love, being met in an experience. This is how grieving and supporting our grief is an act of love, and self-love. Our tears move us *toward* our grief, and *toward* our hearts, so that our tears can flow and our body can let go.

Unwittingly, we hold against our feelings, or feel only "acceptable" feelings, those typically predetermined by our families of origin, in the service of "safety." We can slowly come to know that holding against our feelings is not real safety, but an old safety. We feel disbelief, shock, fear, despair, sadness, regret,

Becoming aware of ourselves and our bodies helps pave the pathway toward an ever-present and ever-deepening connection and intimacy with ourselves and others. This is the nature of true love, being met in an experience. This is how grieving and supporting our grief is an act of love, and self-love. Our tears move us toward our grief, and toward our hearts, so that our tears can flow, and our body can let go.

guilt, and remorse that can feel as if it will never end. It is hard to support these feelings inside of ourselves. We need time and space and help to support these feelings and to allow ourselves to *experience* them as emotions inside the body.

Real safety is having the room to feel the spectrum of our human experience, both light and dark. It can include even being supported in our very human feeling (and *never* the action or deed) of, for example, wanting revenge, hatred, wanting to kill, or wanting to die. These, too, are natural feelings for which we need a connection—another human who can genuinely be with us and say something like "Me too," "I get it. It makes sense you would feel this way," "I'm here," "I know these feelings inside of me and can be here with you as you support them inside of you." When we can support all of our feelings, we will not act out on ourselves or another human being. This is the taking responsibility for our humanity, light and dark. This is part of an inner journey to follow the trail of pain in the body and meet it with kindness and gentleness. It often begins first with being met outwardly by another, in these harder, "darker" feelings, with acceptance. It is not a journey through a dark underworld to somewhere *outside* of yourself. Rather, it is a journey to become deeply acquainted with those energies of the dark underworld in all of us.

This work is not always easy, but it is fruitful. We need guides and elders for safe passage who are the living embodiment of having made it through. How will you know? Your body will tell you. Perhaps there is a guide that comes to mind for you now? For many of us, animals or images from the natural world often feel safer than our fellow humans. For others, we can bring in a person or spirit/source/unconditional love, or wherever you place your faith—inside or outside of you.

Healing trauma in the body after loss is anything but linear, and it can feel slow and confusing. We must respect our organismic nature of moving into expansion and contraction, opening and closing. The nature of psychotherapy is a weekly rhythm of moving toward and away. Coming into connection and going away from connection. This is the rhythm of life. Attachment and detachment. We need support for both experiences, connection and separateness. One of the first things I do with my clients is support and honor their "no" to anything I offer. Any resistance to an embodiment experiment, or to a next step, must be honored so they do not push past or go beyond their supports to gain approval, or to "get somewhere." That pushing past their felt sense of a boundary is often coming from pressure, and pressure can be retraumatizing. When our "no" is honored, we feel safer, our body relaxes, and we can find our way home. This home means back to the body, back to the ground again, and trusting our own knowing with reverence and attunement to our process.

When we lose someone precious to us, our bodies take the hit. How we process that loss physically, emotionally, mentally, and spiritually can feel overwhelming. Grief teaches us powerlessness. All of my work as a psychotherapist includes healing varying degrees of childhood trauma. The reality is that no child has support for their powerlessness. In fact, in order to survive, they must strategically develop coping skills in order to *not* feel their powerlessness. They learn to live on top of a repressed feeling of powerlessness. Therein lies the journey home to our inner children, and all that is unlived in each of us that still needs and deserves expression. Thus, grief becomes an opportunity to recover aliveness within ourselves. With the loss of a loved one, we must turn our gaze inward to the map of the body, to our hearts, and ask: "What is alive for me today, in this moment, in this body?" I invite my clients to move toward a feeling in the body, be with it, perhaps ask it why it is here and what it may need. Does this feeling have a message for you? What is the origin story of this feeling? Let your body speak to you. It may tell you of the decades of shame you carry, the blame, the anger, the agony, or of a legacy of "not enough-ness" that is new or ancient in your generational lineage.

Notes from the Field

Remember, there is nowhere to get as we grieve. We do not need to stop being afraid; we need to let our fear be here, and to reach for and feel support. We do not need to stop being angry. Instead, we need to ground our anger and use it for our lifeforce, not against our life. We are human, and we are enough. Any sense of not enough-ness inside of us is because along the way "it" (support) was not enough. Helping clients to see how they are enough as they grieve whoever they have lost is our work. We need love for the way we all live our loss and heartbreak.

What does it mean to "take in a connection for a feeling"? With the mind, it looks like "Aha, I get it," whereas taking in a connection into the body is different, and subtle, and takes time. I often invite my clients to take in *one drop* of connection from me (or a safe support they were able to conjure) into one cell of their body. I imagine the drop of connection landing right into my client's heart. What does it mean to ground into a feeling? On a body level, I invite my clients to imagine that they are a tree with deep roots. They are bringing the feelings down through their legs and letting their body connect and be supported by the great Mother Earth.

I support my clients in trusting their feelings and noticing whenever a "critical" energy comes in. I encourage them to stay with their perception and their feelings. To the extent that many of us live with even an unconscious distrust of real connection, we "hold out" connection. When working with clients, I will often tell them, "You can distrust me, and I will still be here." I support their inner child's discernment, from way back then, to not trust that their heart could be met the way they need it to be. They distrust that I could know anything about their pain and suffering. I do not need them to know that I do. I need them to feel how their distrust saved their lives. I tell them, "I trust your distrust. I trust your fear or terror. I trust your confusion." Slowly, over time, our relationship creates the container for a glimmer of trust to appear.

Time Is Long and Short and Continuous

After great loss, our lives become delineated into two distinct blocks of time— before the loss and after the loss. We feel at odds with time, and every day that passes is a day farther away from our loved ones. For many of us, we would do anything to go back in time.

There is no "moving on" from grief, only learning to live alongside it and honoring it as our own. We need to give ourselves permission to be [fill in the feeling] for the rest of our lives. With every change, there can be more grief. It is the often-excruciating energetic invitation to return to our hearts. Grief initiates us back to our body, back to love, and into a deeper relationship with spirit/source/unconditional love/nature, and to our own true nature. Pema Chödrön (2016) writes: "The healing comes from letting there be room for all of this to happen: room for grief, for relief, for misery, for joy."

Our old web of connection and the people in it disappear after we lose a loved one. Then something can happen very slowly and over time if we are open to it: a new web appears. People who know what we know and have lived something close to what we have lived through. Surprisingly, there is energetic resonance. It is not often even what we wanted, yet there it is—it is what we have. It is a great mystery of sorts how this happens, but over time, it does. We all participate in this. Hold the vision, trust the process. Our lives have meaning and our hearts matter and can touch people in ways we never could have expected.

Perhaps my deepest offering for meeting our grief when we are alone would be something like this:

Go now to your sofa or bed and feel the softness of your blankets. If it feels right, bring a small pillow to your belly and hold it as though you were holding your inner child. Invite your body to relax. Invite your mind to quiet its chatter and bring your attention to your heart. Become the energy of the mother you had, or wish you had: perhaps calm, tender, confident, openhearted, relaxed, and centered inside herself. Bring whatever mothering image comes to you and imagine being held in a cocoon of love as you cocoon your little you. Feel the great Mother Earth beneath you. All that will come and grow beneath you, and all that has lived before you, composting and renewing, doing what she does. Feel Father Sky above you: the night sky, holding all of the past, all we have loved. Feel how they are still a part of the whole constellation of everything. We are connected to them in this world and the cosmos. Feel the great expanse of time, and timelessness: the past, present, and future, of which you and all of your loved ones are a part. Now imagine, if you can, a hand holding yours, the hand of a loved one, a person, or the presence of an animal, or a tree could be with you or next to you in this cocoon of love. Invite spirit/source/unconditional love in and feel this presence—perhaps in birdsong, sunlight or moonlight, or an image of safety. If spirit/source/unconditional love could speak to you now, what might they say? Perhaps something like: "I've been here all along. I love you." Listen to whatever you hear.

"Give your wounds constant and caring attention," the mythologist Michael Meade (2017) says, "for the essential nature of every human soul is gifted, noble and wounded." Grief is a practice to help us to heal our wounds and our souls. Let your tears, which are in life layer, fall, and let them speak the words of your heart. From there, your healing will ripple and flow into the hearts of others and the heart ocean of the world.

Become willing to accept change, however agonizing. Dedicate your days to self-forgiveness, self-compassion, and self-love. Our egos that were blown open by loss never go down without trying to blame ourselves or others before we step into taking full responsibility for our lives. Only with the wisdom that comes through healing and living past the pain do we lose the line between self and other. The mind is a terrible master. Let your mind follow your heart. As you come to love yourself, you can come to love the world again. This is not easy, but it is possible. This is the spiraling spiritual path.

May you know peace, though war exists. May you know wholeness, though we are all sums of parts. May you trust yourself, your perception, and your body to guide you back to your heart so you can be with it and be it. You deserve your own love and your own aliveness, vitality, realness, and vulnerability, in spite of whatever pain you carry. You deserve to show up as you are, not acting out, and belonging fully. You belong to this world and this world belongs to you. Death is not an ending, though it can feel like it.

May your body sing the songs of sorrow and of beauty, and may you feel the chorus of the earth singing along with you. May you have moments of feeling your truest aliveness, despite painful losses. May you fully inhabit your body and inhabit your life. May you not feel alone but connected to your heart and the heart of everyone and every living thing that has come before you, and who will come after you. And in this moment, may you feel your own breath and life force. May you find a way to metabolize, weave, and dance with your grief. May you discover your True Self.

Love for our lives must include embracing the pureness of our grief. In each moment, our pain, our agony, our joy, our light, our mistakes, our triumphs, our needs, our longings, our gifts, our offerings, our pureness...all of it, right there. All of this is in each breath and in each moment. We step into this moment in the fullness of it all and serve the flow of life itself.

Grief teaches us how to love. All grief is a love story. It teaches us our resilience. With every loss, we learn how to love differently. Our remorse, if there, is always a teacher. Guilt is a gust, sometimes productive, sometimes useless. Remorse, however, is a guide and teacher in how we can grow in our capacity to love. And gratefulness—gratefulness leads to closure (Perls, 1970). Perhaps this is the journey of life, getting to our gratefulness, however unimaginable, implausible, and impossible this may seem.

Loving others can feel like the easy part. Grieving our loved ones brings forward the challenging poignancy and preciousness of life. How do we carry on in love? We feel perhaps an urgency to act in ways we may not have previously. As well, it is the reminder that our time too will come to an end. Life is hard and painful, and it is beautiful and numinous. Grief initiates us to know ourselves, to heal ourselves, to love more deeply, tenderly, and universally. It connects us all. We are all vulnerable and we need one another. May you meet your vulnerability and experience its power. And may you experience the potency of your powerlessness. May you know peace in your heart. May you become a wounded healer. May you be at home in your body. May you be love and a creator of more love and expression. May something new be born from your pain and loss.

Perhaps there is ultimately but one grief and we all share in it. Perhaps there is but one life and we all share in it, and it is the life of the soul, which is eternal. Our unique souls, our unique pain and suffering, here together in this moment, with gratitude, connected to each other and all of life. Here we are together. This moment, where divinity and humanity converge. One.

References

Alpert, S., Lupin-Alpert, N., Hadden, D. & Hadden, S. (2021). *Hartford Family Institute's Professional Training Program Manual: The Study of Body-centered Psychotherapy and Subtle Energy Healing.* West Hartford, CT: HFI.

Chödrön, P. (2016). *When Things Fall Apart: Heart Advice for Difficult Times.* Boulder, CO: Shambhala Press.

Gendlin, E.T. (2007). *Focusing: How to Gain Direct Access to Your Body's Knowledge.* London: Bantam.

Hanh, T.N. [Thích Nhất Hạnh]. (2013, July 29). If you know how to suffer, you suffer less [Video]. YouTube. www.youtube.com/watch?v=DTgv4iPgQ2o

Hanh, T.N. [Thích Nhất Hạnh]. (2015). *The Way Out Is In: The Zen Calligraphy of Thich Nhat Hanh.* London: Thames and Hudson.

Hanh, T.N. [Thích Nhất Hạnh]. (2018, January 14). No birth, No death. YouTube. www.youtube.com/watch?v=G-3O3rG_okc

Kunitz, S. (1971). *The Testing-Tree.* Boston, MA: Little, Brown.

Meade, M. (Producer). (2017). Mosiac Voices [Audio podcast]. www.mosaicvoices.org/living-myth-project

Perls, F.S. (1970). Chapter 2: Four Lectures. In J. Fagan & I.L. Shepherd (eds) *Gestalt Therapy Now: Theory, Techniques, Applications* (pp.14–38). New York, NY: Harper and Row.

Taylor, S.E. (2012). Tend and Befriend Theory. In P.A.M. Van Lange, A.W. Kruglanski & E.T. Higgins (eds) *Handbook of Theories of Social Psychology* (pp.32–49). Thousand Oaks, CA: Sage Publications.

CHAPTER 20

Release to Relief

The Wail of Grief

Deborah Koff-Chapin

I t is so close, so natural, so universal…yet so many of us do not have access to the healing power of our own voices.

I was a freshman in college. A close friend from high school had died instantly in a car accident. I was numb. I did not know how to integrate this—the first death of a friend. Entering the funeral home, I saw her mother. A primal wail began to rise from her body. I began to join her in sorrowful sound. I could finally feel. A wave of relief passed through me as I realized I could immerse myself in shared grief. I was touching into a timeless ritual. Other voices began to join this archetypal human song. There was beauty in giving voice to our sorrow. As the momentum of our communal expression began to grow, the funeral director scurried into the vestibule. I could sense his fear of emotions getting out of control. As he opened the doors and ushered us into the chapel, the plug was pulled from our container. The wave of collective mourning receded. As I sat in the chapel, my numbness returned. The words of the officiant felt like platitudes in the face of the mystery of death. Francis Weller, psychotherapist, grief expert and soul activist, articulates what I was intuiting:

> To be empty, to feel empty, is to live in the wasteland near the gates of death. This is intolerable to the soul. We were not meant to live such shallow lives. Our heritage and our psychic makeup are designed for an elaborate richness of imagination and creativity that allows us to feel intimately connected to the ongoing creation. We were meant to drop below the surface of things and to experience the depths of life in the same ways that our deep-time ancestors did. Their lives were filled with story, ritual, and circles of sharing. Their lives were not shamefully hidden away but known—losses, defeats,

grief, pains, joys, births, deaths, dreams, sorrows; the communal draw of life was open and acknowledged. This is what the soul expected, what it is we need today. (Weller, 2015)

A few years later, I met a woman who created a container that could hold the primal expression I longed for. Inspired by her visits to Pueblo and Ute tribal dances, Elizabeth Cogburn had asked: "Where are our ceremonial dances?" (Cogburn, 1986). In response to this question, she developed a group practice called the *Long Dance*. It was crafted to honor the individualistic psyche of the contemporary Western personality within a unified field. Held by the heartbeat of the drum, participants move and sing within concentric circles to embody different qualities of energy—yin, yang, witness, freeform, contemplative. Each person follows their own impulse while honoring the larger whole of which they are a part. One might be in a deeply internal space while another engaged in comedic play. In my first Long Dance, I felt the safety and spaciousness to open my voice. Deep into the night, I moved rhythmically to the beat of the drum, wailing a primal song. I was embodying the fullness of my soul through ancient yet timeless forms of expression (Cogburn, 1984).

Through the integration of this practice in my life, I was able to trust my voice at another funeral. The news of my cousin's shocking death in an accident reached me on the West Coast. I rushed to the airport to be with family. After the service, we went to his parents' home. I watched my aunt. She was busy being the perfect host. I wondered how she could do this at such a time. I gazed around the room. It looked like a social event. I couldn't help but feel the disparity between surface appearances and the reason we were together. The pressure began to build within me. Feeling compelled to express the underlying intensity of the situation, my body rose up with a force I could not contain. I began to improvise a passionate, mournful cantor-like song. It felt like I was pouring forth the sorrow of the whole group. It was an archetypal expression of grief. I came to completion and sat back down. I had really stepped out of the norm. No one spoke about it to me.

To this day, I have no idea what they thought. On one level I was embarrassed—but I also trusted the authenticity of the impulse, even if it created discomfort in this social setting. I had acted upon my authentic impulse, despite the fact that others could not join me.

Sobonfu Somé, one of the foremost voices in African spirituality to come to the West, shares her perspective:

> It is natural that people around you start to grieve when you do. We know that when you have pain it's not a personal pain, it is a pain of the whole group. We experience a collective sharing, so that an individual doesn't need to bear all the weight of the suffering. (Somé, n.d.)

What has happened to us in contemporary society? How have we lost touch with our natural, human ways? This place of collective grieving provides solace and release. Yet we block it off in fear of...what? When we hide our feelings, we keep them circulating through our bodies, impacting our physical and mental health. And in denying the power of our grief, we also limit our capacity for joy and creativity. Giving voice to feelings is a natural human process. We must regain this human birthright.

Core art forms such as singing, drumming, dancing, and image making emerged in cultures all over the world. They enable us to express, transform, and embody our feelings, to gain insight and renew our vision. Contemporary culture has redirected the arts towards competitive, talent-driven professions. We have abandoned the original role of the arts as essential for a healthy human life. I believe that the burgeoning expressive arts movement is helping us to reclaim the arts for healing, wholing, and inspiring. Integration of the arts into life brings fulfillment and community connection.

We can begin by taking simple steps in our own lives. Our voice is the most basic vehicle of expression we have. Here are some ways of opening to vocal expression. In simply acting, we plant potent seeds.

Breathing to Sighing

Empty your lungs with long slow outbreaths. Notice the fullness of in-breath that is enabled by the depth of your out-breath. Allow the out-breath to become audible. First, emphasize the sound of the air moving through your throat. Gradually, let it vibrate your vocal cords, becoming a sigh. This is a self-care act we do naturally to release stress. When doing this consciously, notice how the sound of your sigh vibrates your chest. Continue this gentle, nurturing sigh for as long as you like. It might even open into a yawn. You can do this any time to offer yourself some loving care.

Opening Your Voice

Once you have allowed sound to flow through sighing, it can be easier to take the next step into a fuller expressive voice. This is something you might like to explore in a private space. Begin with an audible breath and sigh. Allow your breath to vibrate your vocal cords even more fully. You do not have to create a musical tone. Play with your own sound—high, low, rhythmic, arhythmic. Notice how each sound vibrates uniquely in your body. You can shape the sounds through moving your mouth and face, especially using the different vowels. Focus on your felt sense of the vibration in your body rather than what it sounds like to others. At some point a feeling might begin to rise through your voice of its own accord—a wave of anger, sorrow, laughter, or a mixture of feelings might rise through your sound. Trust that this is natural and healthy. If you don't resist, it will come to its own conclusion.

As we provide space for the expression of our feelings, we expand and open to a deeper, timeless aspect of ourselves—our souls. As you open your voice, you may discover beauty as well as pain. Below I offer a range of ways to enrich your vocal explorations.

Toning

Many people have been told not to sing at some point in their childhood. It is amazing the power of one criticism to impact creative expression for the rest of one's life. Toning is a more musical approach to free-form vocalizing. It tends to emerge naturally as long notes created through vowel sounds. (See the section "The Healing Power of the Voice" in Chapter 4.)

Words to Chants

Let a simple word or phrase arise in your mind. You might begin by saying it over and over, until you hear the rhythmic pattern and tune inherent within its sounds. It may begin to sound like a chant or prayer arising from your own psyche. If more words come, give them shape as well. You might like to turn on a recording app in your phone to remember your personal chant.

Movement

It is natural to move with your vocal expression. Standing is conducive to movement, though not necessary. Closing your eyes can help you focus on the unity of your voice and body. You might begin by allowing your hands to express the sounds coming from your voice. Your feet might provide a rhythm or convey you through space. Let your sound inspire your movement. And, in turn, let your voice be impacted by your movement. You are a unified being and all the art forms spring from the same source.

Simple Instruments

A musical instrument can create a platform upon which to vocalize. You do not have to be a trained musician to have the satisfaction of playing an instrument. There are many simple and affordable instruments. All you need is one instrument to open a new path in your vocal explorations.

RHYTHMIC INSTRUMENTS

- These are the most universal and archetypal instruments. The beat of our hearts provides a constant, though little noticed, rhythm in our lives. A drum or rattle can be all you need to dive deep into meditative sound.
- A rattle is a container with small items inside. When shaken, it creates an oddly satisfying sound. Rattles are made from dried gourds, shaped leather, carved wood, shells, or formed plastic. The easiest way to make a rattle is to put beans, seeds, or stones inside a small closable jar.
- Most cultures have drums of some kind. Some are beaten with sticks and others with the hands. A music store or online search can show you a range of possibilities. It is best to try out a drum before buying it, to sense its rightness for you. There are also drum-making workshops that can give you a more personal connection with your drum.
- Whether using a rattle or drum, you can simply play until you settle into a hypnotic rhythm. This provides its own satisfaction and can support inner imagery or journeying. Let your voice be carried along with the shake of your rattle or the pulse of your drum.
- Rhythmic instruments allow us to settle into alignment with the pulse of life and oneness with the earth.

TONAL INSTRUMENTS

Though many tonal instruments require long study to master, there are some that are easily played. They might hold a single note or allow for multiple chords.

- Singing bowls can be made of a mixture of metals, like Himalayan bowls or Buddhist temple bowls. Contemporary versions of both are available online and in metaphysical shops. These bowls tend to have a complex harmonics. Crystal singing bowls are a recent invention and use high-tech glass. There notes are purer and more piercing in tone. You can play any singing bowl in two ways. Striking it with a suede stick enables strong percussive notes. Rubbing the rim with the stick allows a smooth, held tone. You can combine bowls to create chords.
- Singing bowls have a celestial sound quality that can inspire a sense of connection with the cosmos.

CHORDAL INSTRUMENTS

Chordal instruments can help us find the songs of our souls. Chordal in-struments can be complex to learn, but there are some that are accessible.

- An autoharp is a stringed instrument that has buttons. Each button mutes all the notes but the ones in its stated chord. All you need to do is press a button and strum!
- A shruti box requires the pumping of air through a book-like box. Different notes and chords can be sustained through continuous pumping.
- Kalimba and mbira are related instruments. They are sometimes called thumb pianos. While gripping the wooden structure in your hands, you can strike metal bars with your thumbs to create rhythmic tonal patterns.
- Ukuleles are small guitar-like instruments that have become popular. The small neck and four strings make for easier chording than a guitar.

This is by no means a complete list of instruments that can be easily played, but it demonstrates the range of possibilities and inspires you to explore how you can create a mesmerizing sound field that supports you to also open your voice.

Music in Nature

Singing and playing while immersed in nature can be deeply healing. It can bring you into relationship with specific life forms—a tree in your yard or a body of water near your home. Breathing deeply as you vocalize, you can fill with the fragrance of your surroundings. It can help expand our sense of communion with something larger. It can also be a time of expressing our love and grief for the earth in these intensifying times of climate change. I do believe that our music can be felt and heard by nature. It is a way to reach out and beyond our human identity to expand our relationship with life. This, in itself, is a healing service for the planet.

Group Vocalizing, Instrumentalizing, and Moving

So now we come full circle. I recall those early lonely experiences—my wailing cries silenced in the funeral home—and later, when I was able to trust my own voice, being the lone expressor of feelings within a group of mourners. Since inviting a few friends to join me in the long dance 40 years ago, I have had a circle of safety and connection for my soul. We have danced, drummed, and sung together through parenting, eldering, and dying (Koff-Chapin, 1983).

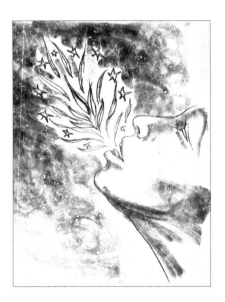

You, too, can plant the seeds of authentic, soulful, and, might I say, sacred arts in your life. Simply invite others to join you. In gathering with a group to drum, rattle, sing, and move, we begin to generate a sense of soul community. We learn to be authentic with one another. And in times of need, we have the vehicles of expression to support each other in grief—bringing beauty and sacredness into the challenging times of our lives.

References

Cogburn, E. (1984). Warriors of the beauty way: Realizing the power of human potential by creating in beauty. An interview with Elizabeth Cogburn by Ross Chapin. *Art and Ceremony in Sustainable Culture*, Spring. www.context.org/iclib/ic05/cogburn

Cogburn, E. (1986, December). New song dance. *New Song Journal*, 4(2). Private newsletter.

Koff-Chapin, D. (1983). Living with Ceremonial and Finding Depth. *In Context: Being a Planetary Villager*, December. www.context.org/iclib/ic01/chapin

Somé, S. (n.d.). Embracing grief: Surrendering to your sorrow has the power to heal the deepest of wounds. Sobunfu Some. www.sobonfu.com/articles/writings-by-sobonfu-2/embracing-grief

Weller, F. (2015*). The Wild Edge of Sorrow: Rituals of Renewal and the Sacred Work of Grief*. Berkeley, CA: North Atlantic Books.

CHAPTER 21

Celebration

Navigating Clients Through the Objects of a Family
Loss, and as Transgenerational Experience
Yon Walls

To feel our grief is innate, yet in most Western societies, we have to get permission to feel, and grief is no exception. Perhaps it's not until we experience grief that we understand the conditioning of emotional expression in our culture, and for sure we come to the insight that speaking with someone honestly about our feelings and being heard related to grief is a unique and *inward* relational experience. By contrast:

> Today, when nearly every question can be handled instantly by Siri, or Google or Alexa, we're losing the habit of pausing to look inward, or to one another, for answers. But even Siri doesn't know everything. And Google can't tell you why your son or daughter is feeling hopeless or excited, or why your significant other feels not so significant lately, or why you can't shake that chronic low-level anxiety that plagues you. (Brackett, 2019)

It also can't tell you what that generational angst is—the feeling that something big or more subtle epigenetically happened before you were born generations ago in your family. And yes, that includes the human experience of grief. We learn how to grieve along the path of our present life and development, including ancestral ways that went before. Perhaps a goal after one's loss and grieving is to experience our way of grief with greater insights and a sense of continuation that speaks to one's ancestral identity and celebration.

And when the grief process has taken its natural course, a private creative celebration that culminates in the joy to be alive can be accomplished by a client's gratefulness to be thawed from the winter of her/his grief and discovering a new relationship to and with the *objects* of the beloved. As grief is a natural process, unlike depression or anxiety, the celebratory process of grief can be organically realized, especially if one isn't hampered by specific cultural expectations of grief. Finding solace through our religious and/or spiritual practices can hold great value, or we can create a new practice and/or ritual for celebration.

Nobel Prize-winning author Orhan Pamuk and his novel *The Museum of Innocence* (2008), perhaps more than any one single factor, contributed to the healing of my personal grief after my mother's death and allowed me to celebrate her life and legacy with a relationship to her physical possessions. It is not only what she owned but what she loved, who she knew, her interests, stages of life, and more expressed through her objects of possession. Losing my mother just after the announcement of the Covid-19 pandemic in the United States, my need to know and possess items that she knew and had lived with was great. Pamuk's novel brilliantly tells a love story and the aftermath of a man's life through the collection and final public display of his beloved girlfriend's possessions; through the process, he comes to terms with her loss and his complicated grieving.

Sometimes our clients need us as companions of their grief to discover their loved one's possessions, not as simple things but objects that possess meaning—the things that we almost desire to speak to us, to tell us a hidden story about the person we loved and lost to death. These objects take on new meaning and in alchemical ways reconnect us to our loved one and transport us therapeutically to nurturing memories every time we encounter the object. That hair comb, favorite tee shirt, a stone acquired from a faraway place, a seashell, a chair, or favorite book, all speak a story and become a kind of talisman for helping to heal the grief. The objects can also become a gateway for celebration of one's past, present, and future as a transgenerational individual or family experience. Death is a universal human experience that knows no boundaries.

Guiding clients to discover and/or rename objects that honor the client's spiritual connection to a loved one can be the intervention that aids the natural grief process. Remember, the object has no true meaning simply as an object, but becomes an object of meaning related to one's connection to the loved one! The client's desire to select and story-tell about an object for self and/or for others is the first step for getting the client to a place of reverence and peace of the lost loved one.

Intervention #1: The Celebratory Storytelling Object

An object of the one lost and loving that object/thing can be profoundly supportive, or a kind touchstone when needed. "We learn to feel a sense of a heart connection in experiences of praise and grief...when we love the things we have, it is called praise, when we love what is lost, it is called grief" (Lowenstal, 2004, p.1245).

Finding or recreating a story related to a loved one's once-owned object can be the resource of solace that's turned to again and again. The first principle that serves the practitioner in this process and intervention is guidance for the client with curious exploration versus needing to be the expert. Empathically being present for the client and listening to his/her journey to find an object is the task. Following the client's emotional resonance related to an object is the start.

First, have the client find or locate an object that they feel close to and that always reminds them of their loved one. This process may happen very quickly or may take several days, or even weeks. It should be an organic process that invites the client to explore a concrete object, or several before choosing one, in which the heart, mind, body, and intuition leads.

Finally, after the client finds an object, giving it a story to keep for self and/or for sharing with others is the intention. It is in attaching a story to the object that it is imbued with greater meaning related to the one loss which can bring joy and reverence that is full of energy and a vibrant sense of continuation and celebration.

Remembering

Sometimes after a long grieving period, the act of remembering—putting together parts of an experience again related to an object—returning to the experience, can be difficult, or not so clear. Yet allowing oneself to find an object through a process of re-*membering* can be a powerful revelation. Engaging an object once held by the beloved that leads one back to an experience (real or imagined) held by the beloved, or perhaps one already in one's possession by the beloved, can be celebratory. It can finally provide one with the spiritual and/or emotional clarity of the loss for greater meaning and resilience and preserve the accomplishments, gifts, and unique contributions of a family's descent. A selected celebratory object (or one that selects you) can be joyous and invigorating as a personal and transpersonal experience.

It can offer one the insights into humanity's experience of death, loss, and transformation for continuation.

Intuition

According to author and leading intuition scholar Shakti Gawain (n.d.), "Every time you don't follow your inner guidance, you feel a loss of energy, loss of power, a sense of spiritual sadness." The intuitive approach allows the client to follow their inner guidance and to feel *into* an object that speaks to their grief. Invite the client to choose a time of day or a specific season to consider an object for celebration.

Inheritance

With this approach, the object for celebration is something that is intentionally and often lovingly left behind specifically for a loved one, and especially revered or possessed for its value identified by the deceased. Also, by the nature of inheritance, it can be viewed as a transpersonal object in that it held perhaps another worldly quality for the beloved.

A Moving Pod

Sometimes there are objects that need to be given away or discarded for discovery of the most important object left by the deceased. This is an intervention that I developed for clients when assisting my own daughter through her grief process after losing a life partner of over a decade to the Covid-19 virus. During her grieving period, she found it difficult to move physically and spiritually from the physical location where she had lived with her partner, and wasn't able to actually start the process of moving her belongings from her home to a new address until after the purchase of a portable moving and storage pod. The pod allowed her to selectively transition items from the home into the pod storage (in what I describe as a *transitional space*) that held her emotional process until she was able to move her objects/items from the pod (left in her driveway) to the actual new location. It is in this transitional space and time that a celebrated object of her lost one was discovered.

The Storytelling Object

After the object has been identified, have the client, in a spontaneous storytelling style, tell you about the object. It may be something already told to the client by the loved one, or perhaps fragments of an incomplete story related to the object. It's important not to overthink it. If they struggle with telling a story, have them create one of their own based on their experience and/or reception of the object! In Pamuk's novel, his lost love leaves behind an earring that indelibly reminds him of their romantic beginning. Years after her death, he is transported by the object that holds a myriad of stories of their life together.

Once the client's story has been told or created and is fairly clear in the client's mind, guide the client to consider the object as one of *celebration*. The concept of celebration can be described as one in which the client has met most of the hardships of grief, denial, and finally acceptance of the loss. At this juncture in the process of grief, a new door has opened toward one's future, and what has been left behind can be celebrated on a personal level, as well as a spiritual and/or transpersonal one. This may be a time when the one left behind can more clearly see their path as generational, and the gift of the beloved is a symbol of ancestral resilience, hope, loyalty, creativity, prosperity, or a special talent. Once the object is or can be envisioned as an object of celebration, the client can choose to create a special place for it, or a place where it can easily be accessed as a memory resource. Also, at various times of year or seasons, a private special happening can be created to celebrate memory of the object. A dance under the moon, a special meal, listening to a favorite song, or a long walk are just some of the ways to celebrate the object of the beloved.

More About Naming an Object

Naming the object is an option for a client if desired. The client shouldn't be pressured or required to name an object of a loved one lost. However, naming an object can enhance the ritual of remembrance.

Intervention #2: Family-Made Group Watercolor Painting

A collective family gathering and painting of an object that acknowledges historical trauma and/or the loss of a loved family member can be an effective activity for creating a memorable object for the entire family created by the family. A grander public example of this kind of art activity (yet very personal to families) is now displayed in and around Ground Zero and across New York City commemorating the 9/11 attacks. Various children's messages and images created by family members of lost loved ones can be seen by the public everyday as a show of remembrance of the collective trauma. In a clinical context, this activity is most suited for clients and/or family members who have accepted the loss and have completed the early season of grief.

Materials and Method
- Large pieces of watercolor paper (as large as available) or butcher paper
- Watercolor paints and large watercolor paintbrushes
- Large plastic water cups and paper towels, water
- Large-tip black Sharpies.

Once materials have been gathered, decide on a day and time for individuals to gather to paint. The painting time should be spontaneous and the group planner should express to participants that knowing how to draw or paint is not required! The only requirement is the group's desire to freely and honestly express through watercolor and markers by writing something about the lost loved one. Watercolor as a specific medium of expression is preferred, as the medium by its nature allows emotions through color to be rendered more easily and flexibly. It is suggested that everyone paints at the same time, allowing a spontaneous depiction of whatever emerges in the moment, including written words and messages. The watercolor image created with language creates a kind collage of varied images and language. Afterwards, the group can decide how the image will be shared and/or displayed and where.

References

Brackett, M. (2019). *Permission to Feel: Unlocking the Power of Emotions to Help Our Kids, Ourselves, and Our Society Thrive*. New York: Celedon Books.

Gawain, S. (n.d.). Quotes. www.goodreads.com/quotes/186604-every-time-you-don-t-follow-your-inner-guidance-you-feel

Lowenstal, M. (2004). *Alchemy of the Soul: The Eros and Psyche Myth as a Guide for Transformation*. Berwick, ME: Nicolas-Hays.

Pamuk, O. (2008). *The Museum of Innocence*. New York, NY: Alfred A. Knopf.

June Morning in April

I thought of you this morning
watching the dark night fade
and merge with the pale dawn

I thought of how you took
a ragged seed and planted it
in a field of fallow dreams

where now

  a blue violet

    grows

      between the

        stones

~ Steven "Mud" Roues

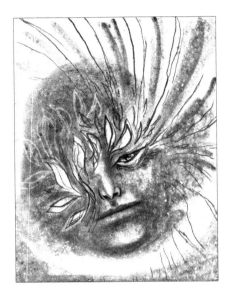

Conclusion

Claudia Coenen

Human beings have evolved through sparks of creativity, leaps of imagination and flashes of insight. Of all mammalian species, we have the unique ability to forge connections and to innovate through our understanding of these connections whether they are to other people, to animals or to our natural surroundings. We also are beings with big emotions and can be shaken and shattered by events in our lives. Creative thinking, expressive processes and therapeutic methods tap into our personal resilience and ingenuity, offering the possibility for healing and growth.

As a teenager, I engaged in an airmail discussion with my great-aunt Hilde, who lived in France after escaping the Nazis in WWII. I asserted that every person is creative. Hilde, a free spirit despite her upbringing, disagreed, saying that only some people were creative. Hilde was correct in her view that only rare (and lucky) artists are truly great; she was thinking of Miro, Picasso, Hemingway, Balanchine. I was saying that we all are able to think differently, to create little gems of pleasure, expression and beauty, without necessarily trying to become a famous and recognized artistic luminary. Aunt Hilde was talking about a product or goal. I was referring to process. I still believe that my definition of creativity, something every human innately has inside, is the "right" one. Using a creative process when one is deeply grieving really does work.

Each of the writers in this book speaks in their own voice from the depths of their own life experiences. We have experienced profound losses that have shaped our lives and led us to the work we do in the world and the perspectives we share with our clients, our students and our close ones. We have taken our grief and drawn it into our hearts where it can inform our ability to resonate with those who seek our help and even those we might randomly share a conversation with. We hope the stories and methods within these pages resonate with you and inform your own approach to grief—whether it is affecting a person you work with or yourself.

When I conceived this book, I wanted to collaborate with people who understand grief and have different ways of explaining, approaching and processing it. We live thousands of miles apart, in different time zones and different countries, but the pandemic has connected us through the internet, allowing us to gather in real time, discussing our ideas and our progress. Our "Wisdom Circles," with our faces in little squares on our individual screens, allowed us to encourage and inspire each other. We truly felt that we were collaborating and working on this project together.

I am in awe that these wise individuals have joined me in producing this book. We recognize that not every concept or suggestion will work for everyone because we know that every grief is unique to the circumstance, place and time in which it occurs.

Acknowledgments

Thank you to the amazing writers, who generously shared their expertise and wisdom. Thank you in particular to Bob Neimeyer for being so generous with his time and wisdom. Thank you to my two Deborahs, who have encouraged my whole life and who jumped on board this project from the beginning. Deborah Koff-Chapin's soulful art connects us to sources we are sometimes barely aware of, and I am so grateful for her contributions to this book. We have shared a love of creativity ever since we first danced together when I was three years old. Deborah Mesibov and I have been playing in the tall grasses of life since we were four.

Thank you to the Portland Institute for Loss and Transition for providing a unique learning space so that I might continue to grow as a grief counselor and for inviting me in as guest faculty. Thank you to my colleagues who bolster me when a difficult death comes along. We try to respond to our grieving clients with our whole hearts, yet this can be challenging at times.

Thanks to generations of humans who have lived, loved and lost and who felt, thought and expressed their experiences in poetry, dance, art and prose. Thanks to the researchers who investigate how we experience bereavement and seek to clarify and refine ways to assist.

Thanks to my editor at Jessica Kingsley Publishers, Elen Griffiths, who is always supportive and encouraging. Gratitude to my amazing clients who struggle with their grief and share their suffering and stories with me. Many thanks to my family, especially my sisters, Jenny and Maggie, who listen to me process my work, my ideas and my ongoing grief and rarely tell me to be quiet although they may roll their eyes occasionally.

I need to offer gratitude to my second husband, Moke Mokotoff, who nurtured me with compassion and love for 16 years. Moke became ill as this book was coming together and died shortly after the manuscript was submitted. Love expands our hearts and mine is full.

A special thanks to all of you reading this book. May you take these creative interventions into your own practice, whether it be to draw your feelings, move your own grief or walk on a beach or in a forest, gathering stones, leaves and feathers. May you honor your own losses as you listen to others. May our words, poetry, art and heartfelt suggestions bring you comfort on your own path.

Signs

Longing for a sign
    Reaching towards
No thing
    I feel a tingle in my hair
       (is that you?)

I know you are no longer here

    yet I feel a pull
      at the top
    of my head
(are you there?)

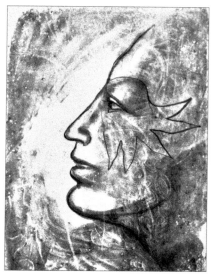

I am haunted sometimes
as I embrace life
    as I engage with
love and song and food, joy and love again

Still I am unmoored

    by your absence

where did you go?
    why are you tugging on my hair?

then I whisper
    as I touch the spot you pulled

       hello.

~ Claudia Coenen

Author Biographies

Claudia Coenen, CGC, FT, MTP, GTMR, is a certified grief counselor in private practice in Hudson, New York, and Fellow in Thanatology. Her books and creative tools help clients process grief and are beneficial to other practitioners. Claudia speaks about creativity and grief at conferences, mental health clinics and hospitals. Claudia has a Masters in Transpersonal Psychology and a certificate in Grief Therapy as Meaning Reconstruction from the Portland Institute where she is a guest lecturer. www.thekarunaproject.com

Kenneth J. Doka, PhD, is Senior Vice-President for the Hospice Foundation of America and Professor Emeritus of The College of New Rochelle. He has authored or edited more than 40 books and more than 100 articles and book chapters. Dr. Doka is editor of *Omega: The Journal of Death and Dying* and *Journeys: A Newsletter to Help in Bereavement*, and has won numerous awards for his work in thanatology. https://drkendoka.com

Robert A. Neimeyer, PhD, directs the Portland Institute for Loss and Transition, practices as a trainer, consultant and coach, and has published more than 600 articles and 35 books, most on grieving as a meaning-making process. He has been awarded Lifetime Achievement Awards by both the Association for Death Education and Counseling and the International Network on Personal Meaning. www.portlandinstitute.org

Louise Allen is an indoor and outdoor integrative counselor and workshop facilitator. Based in and around Faversham, in the South East of England, Louise incorporates inspiration from nature's cycles and processes into her therapeutic work. She co-founded the Faversham Death Café, a relaxed community space to discuss death and dying. www.ferncounselling.space

Sharon Strouse, MA, ATR-BC, LCPAT, is an art therapist and Associate Director of the Portland Institute for Loss and Transition. Her private practice and national presentations on traumatic loss, suicide bereavement and military loss are grounded in meaning reconstruction, continuing bonds and restorative retelling. She has authored many articles, chapters and *Artful Grief: A Diary of Healing*, written 12 years after her daughter's suicide. www.artfulgrief.com

Sarah Vollmann, MPS, ATR-BC, LICSW, is a registered, board-certified art therapist, a Licensed Independent Clinical Social Worker and a faculty member of the Portland Institute for Loss and Transition. She maintains a private practice with a specialization in bereavement and is an author and presenter both nationally and internationally. www.complexloss.com

Catharine DeLong, CM-Th, is a certified music thanatologist, hospice interfaith chaplain, composer and writer. She tends to the emotional, physical and spiritual needs of palliative patients and their families with harp and voice, delivers remote music sessions to isolated patients (Harps of Comfort) and creates original harp scores for audiovisual meditations (Colors in Motion). Catharine lectures on end-of-life issues focusing on music as medicine. Her 2021 video performance at the edge of the Great Salt Lake brings awareness to climate thanatology in collaboration with SixtyEight Art Institute, Copenhagen. www.delongharp.com

Steven "Mud" Roues, published poet and active musician, has appeared with many musical luminaries, including John Lee Hooker, Luther Allison, Carl Perkins, Vassar Clements, Bo Diddley, Lenny Kaye, Wayne Kramer (MC5), B.B. King, Howlin' Wolf, James Cotton, Sam and Dave, and Wilson Pickett. Steven played virtuoso harmonica in Peter Schickele's Lincoln at Ease and The House of The Blues. Bands: Roues Brothers, Finn and the Sharks, UpSouth Twisters, Big Jim Wheeler, Jon Pousette-Dart, and Aztec Two-Step 2.0.

Oceana Sawyer is an end-of-life doula and grief guide, focused on the liminal space of dying, grieving, pleasure and liberation in an eco-somatic context. Her book *Life, Death, Grief and the Possibility of Pleasure* is available now online at Kizzy's Books & More. www.oceanaendoflifedoula.com/patreon

Evie Lindemann, ATR-BC, ATCS, LMFT, is a board-certified art therapist and a licensed marriage and family therapist with Jungian training. She is Associate Professor Emerita at Albertus Magnus College and has exhibited nationally and internationally as a printmaking artist. She has written multiple book chapters and journal articles on grief, loss, spirituality and the expressive arts. She receives inner guidance from her spiritual teacher, Meher Baba, an Indian mystic who maintained silence for 43 years. www.evielindemann.com

Heather Stang, MA, C-IAYT, is the author of *Mindfulness & Grief* and the guided journal *From Grief to Peace*. She is the founder of the Mindfulness & Grief Institute, where she facilitates Awaken, a mindfulness-based online grief group, offers individual sessions and hosts the Mindfulness & Grief Podcast.

Yon Walls, PhD, MFA, MA, is an arts adventurer, lover of the natural world and creative writer from a very early age. These areas of life focus led to her present work as an associate psychotherapist, life coach, published creative writer and a PhD in Psychology. She works with individuals, couples and families from holistic approaches which includes creativity, connection to the natural world, spirituality and historical trauma as potential for transformation.

Deborah Koff-Chapin, BFA, creates her evocative images through the process of Touch Drawing, which she originated in 1974. She teaches the process internationally. Deborah is creator of *SoulCards* 1 and 2, *Portals of Presence* and *SoulTouch Coloring Journals* and author of *Drawing Out Your Soul*. She now holds online Touch Drawing workshops and Song Bath Sanctuary. https://touchdrawing.com

Dorit Netzer, PhD, ATR-BC, LCAT, is an art therapist (www.doritnetzer.com), who is working with families through creative expression, therapeutic play, poetry, mental imagery and dreams. For 25 years, as researcher and educator, Dorit has published on the role of creative expression in health, inquiry and transformative education. https://longisland.academia.edu/DoritNetzer

Ilana (Nancy) Rowe, PhD, REAT, writes, teaches, designs curriculum and leads workshops in transpersonal psychology, creativity, teacher education, spirituality, dream work, imagination and earth-based spirituality at Sofia University. She is semi-retired and balances professional life with an active creative life. She is well published as an academic scholar and has written a memoir about caregiving her husband through his end of life, called *Sacred Stories: A Caregiver's Journey Through Alzheimer's*.

Elizabeth Coplan is a playwright, producer, director, author, and screenwriter. Her nonprofit Grief Dialogues uses art to start conversations about dying, death and grief. Her playwriting credits include the award-winning *Hospice: A Love Story* and *Untold*, one mother's story of stillbirth. Her play *Over My Dead Body* is currently in Off-Broadway development. She is a podcast creator and co-host, the director/producer of several award-winning films and screenwriter/producer of *Honoring Choices*, premiered in Los Angeles in September 2022 at the Reimagine festival. https://griefdialogues.com

Topaz Weis, REACE®, is a registered expressive arts consultant/educator, Founder of Expressive Arts Burlington, LLC, Co-Chair of IEATA's REACE® Professional Standards Committee, a SoulCollage® Facilitator, speaker, astrologer and mother. She serves an international clientele in person and via Zoom, leading people in fun and profound experiences to engage their imaginations and explore their creativity. Topaz's one-on-one expressive arts facilitation, group and organizational workshops, trainings and retreats refresh the spirit and grant new and exciting pathways towards growth and wholeness. https://expressiveartsburlington.com

Deborah Mesibov, BFA, is an artist, designer and poet. As a graphic designer, her career spanned decades in business and corporate environments. Now retired, Deborah currently serves the disability community in job development. She is a lifelong writer.

Becky Sternal, PsyD, LCSW, RSMT, is a somatic psychotherapist specializing in complex PTSD/developmental trauma, depression, anxiety, sexual trauma, grief and intergenerational trauma. She uses somatic techniques, EMDR, parts work, psychedelic integration and breathwork to guide clients in reconnecting with their body's wisdom and inner intelligence to create powerful healing. Email: hudsonpractice@gmail.com

Additional Resources

Alexandra Kennedy, MA, MFT—www.alexandrakennedy.com

Association for Death Education and Counseling—www.adec.org

The Mindfulness & Grief Podcast—https://mindfulnessandgrief.com/grief-podcast

Center for Touch Drawing—https://touchdrawing.com

Surviving the Tsunami of Grief—www.tsunamiofgrief.com

Grief Dialogues: Out of Grief Comes Art Podcast Series—https://griefdialogues.podbean.com

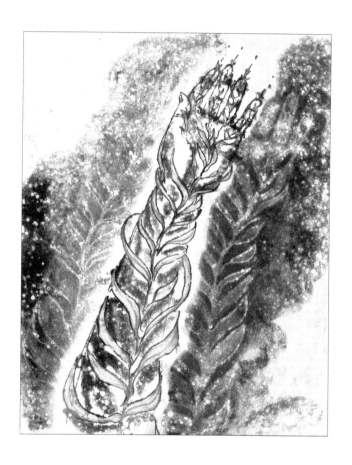

Index